Sleep

ANTI-AGING SLEEP
SECRETS

James W. Forsythe M.D., H.M.D.

Anti-Aging Sleep Secrets

Century Wellness Publishing

Copyright © 2013, By James W. Forsythe, M.D., H.M.D.

All Rights Reserved, including the right of
reproduction in whole or in part in any form.

Forsythe, James W. M.D., .M.D.

Book Design: Patty Atcheson Melton

1. Health   2. Sleep

.

ISBN:978-0-9848383-8-7

Table of Contents

Dedication

I would like to acknowledge Patricia Atcheson Melton
And Wayne Rollan Melton
For their vision, dedication, and hard work in
the creation of this book

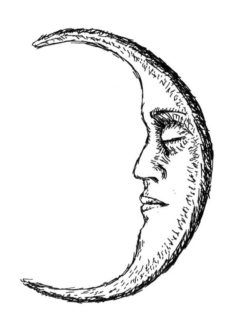

Foreword

By
James W. Forsythe, M.D., H.M.D.

Beauty Sleep Permeates Life

People who fail to get adequate sleep invariably look older than their actual age.

Intense medical research has shown similar results among people of all age groups.

This means that the age-old term of "beauty sleep" or "sleeping beauty" actually has scientific validity.

For you, the question might emerge: "Am I aging too fast due to a lack of sufficient sleep? How much high-quality sleep do I need to look younger?"

To set the groundwork for potential answers, consider a study conducted by Swedish researchers, as reported in the December 14, 2010 issue of the "*British Medical Journal*."

Twenty-three women and men ages 18 through 31 were tested by the researchers in an attempt to chronicle any impact on physical attractiveness from sleep deprivation.

After sleeping for eight hours these people were photographed by researchers. During subsequent nights similar snapshots were taken of these individuals following nights where they experienced little or no sleep. In order to increase the legitimacy of eventual results researchers insisted during the entire study period that these people refrain from wearing make-up and avoid combing their hair.

Later, after researchers finished taking these photographs at the end of each phase of the study, they mixed up the photos almost as if shuffling a deck of cards.

Then, the study team showed these snapshots to 65 people who had not previously participated in the research project. Those who viewed the photograph rated each snapshot on whether they perceived the person as looking healthy, tired or attractive.

Perhaps generating little surprise among seasoned health experts, those viewing the photos considered people as looking less attractive, more tired and less healthy than they appeared following a night of good sleep.

Catch Your Beauty Sleep

"All sleep is 'beauty sleep,'" I sometimes tell patients. "Adding to the proverbial magic, the entire process is free, particularly in healthy people."

Naturally, adequate amounts of high-quality sleep can and should be incorporated into any anti-aging regimen.

This can emerge as particularly important among people who want to prevent, stop or lessen the progression of the natural wrinkling of the skin. Among sleep's many anti-aging benefits:

Moisturizing: As we sleep the body naturally generates "slumber perspiration" that helps moisturize the skin.

Position: Most people sleep lying down, a position that increases vital blood flow to the face—potentially lessening wrinkles while increasing muscle tone.

Rejuvenation: Human growth hormones produced naturally

within the body during healthy sleep repair or alleviate damage to the organs and to the skin.

Ultimately, our bodies generally yearn to remain alive and as youthful for as long as possible. For specific reasons that remain mysterious and difficult to pinpoint among researchers, nature has developed a system that requires a person to experience good sleep in order to thrive.

Essential Questions Arise

Although doctors and many of their patients realize the importance of sleep and its anti-aging qualities, then why do people experience age-related signs such as wrinkling and crumpling bodies?

Certainly to proclaim that sleep serves as a cure-all for any and all ailments or that it guarantees a longer life in every instance would be a tremendous disservice to the public.

Yet for those of us fully cognizant of the significant benefits that sleep can instill, the need to continually and predictably get healthy levels of that activity remains essential.

Herein you'll soon find many of the most significant and primary reasons why we sleep, plus details on the various disorders that curtail, prevent or hamper this activity.

The many pitfalls of inadequate sleep and the benefits of getting high-quality rest will become apparent once you discover the hidden triggering factors or causes involved.

The Essence of Life

In a nutshell, everything comes down to the fact that studies intrinsically prove:

Death: Inadequate sleep can lead to premature aging and even an early end to life.

Life: Good-quality sleep at healthful, non-excessive levels can generate precursors to extended life, a slowdown of the aging process and improved mental capacity.

Moods: The good moods that healthful, natural sleep often makes possible clears the way for positive outlooks on life that can lead to vibrancy and mental sharpness. Conversely, insufficient or disturbed sleep can ignite irritability and grogginess, increasing stress factors that are known to degrade overall health.

Quality: Insufficient or sporadic sleep can wreak havoc on the overall quality of life, disrupting schedules, damaging the ability to focus well on particular topics and potentially leading to a gradual downfall of the internal organs. By contrast, many people who enjoy good sleep feel and benefit from adequate amounts of physical and mental energy. This, in turn opens up a proverbial door to the possibilities life can present.

Essential Goals Emerge

When learning specifics on these various issues and benefits, you'll also discover the basic essentials on how, where and when to strive for the most healthful sleep.

Added importance also hinges on the best, most natural substances—if any—to take in order to induce healthful and deep levels of this essential activity.

Many readers likely will become mesmerized by the discovery and compelling explanations of the many natural strategies of inducing sleepiness. In many instances or the first time in their lives, some people take joy in learning and engaging in these easy-to-understand instructions.

Ample feelings of joyfulness also often emerge from sleep-issue sufferers who learn that they are not alone in their distress and frustrations in finding a "cure."

Also, without a doubt, lots of these individuals appreciate the fact that scientists have pinpointed many of the most integral and natural remedies possible.

Equal emphasis gets placed on the numerous dangerous and highly addictive drugs that some doctors recklessly prescribe in futile efforts to address symptoms of inadequate sleep. Patients worldwide benefit greatly when understanding the specifics of the various types of drug category, plus the dangers imposed by each segment of pills.

Understandably, other essentials focus on how to kick the use of addictive sleeping pills, ways to avoid taking such pharmaceuticals, and the critical need to understand the many drawbacks of all sleep drug categories—sold over-the-counter or by prescription.

Patients Appreciate Natural Sleep Aids

As one of only a handful of licensed integrative medical oncologists in the United States, I often hear patients proclaim how thankful they are to benefit from natural remedies. Now with nearly 50 years of medical practice, I've seen natural substances rather than man-made drugs work wonders for many patients, particularly when issues involve serious sleep problems.

An exceedingly rare practitioner of both natural homeopathy and of so-called standard medicine as well, I've personally witnessed the deadly ravages of powerful sleep drugs—plus the incalculable, endless positive results that natural remedies generate.

Any in-depth discussion of how to address sleep challenges must include a thorough listing and analysis of beneficial natural sleep aids. To do otherwise, to avoid mention or describing these formidable options would be disservice to the public.

Thus, I've included a comprehensive listing of some of the most effective sleep treatments. Many of them are available primarily through homeopaths or other practitioners of natural medicine.

For many patients suffering chronic and potentially life-altering sleep issues, the discovery and use of such natural treatments can bring new hope that they haven't had for many years.

Excellent Results Often Emerge

Without exaggeration, hope springs eternal for lots of patients who start sleeping well for the first time in many years upon taking natural sleep remedies.

Humbled and delighted by their laudatory comments, while approaching my golden anniversary as a health care professional I often hear patients proclaim: "Doctor Forsythe, you look at least 10 or 15 years younger than your actual age."

If time and our particular situation at any given moment permits, I sometime answer honestly and fully that a commitment to healthful sleep can go a long way toward achieving our anti-aging goals.

Along with the many other healthy lifestyle choices that I mention in one of my other hot-selling books, "Your Secret to the Fountain of Youth, What they Don't Want You to Know About HGH," I also benefit from legal injectable natural human growth hormone.

Every week people from across the United States and from around the world visit my Century Wellness Clinic in Reno, Nevada. Patients make these lengthy treks seeking diagnosis and treatment for a variety of ailments, primarily cancer or other health issues as well including bothersome sleep problems.

Through the decades I've literally helped or treated tens of thousands of patients. Those suffering from sleep issues deserve and need serious medical care, although the vast majority of people throughout society apparently remain unaware of the critical nature of such issues.

1
Discover the Anti-Aging Benefits of Napping

Studies consistently show that people enjoy the longest life expectancies in societies where almost everyone takes an afternoon nap.

Countries or regions where people live the longest include the Okinawa islands and Mediterranean nations like Greece, areas where naps are the norm, according to the World Health Organization.

Interestingly, research shows that people from countries where naps are traditional throughout society have longer average life expectancies. This is compared to the shorter life spans on average among overall populations from nations or regions where naps are discouraged, overlooked or frowned upon.

Some physicians also believe that so-called non-traditional diets consisting primarily of healthy foods usually prevail in countries where naps are encouraged.

In the United States, where society discourages or even prohibits naps, the bulk of foods eaten throughout society are generally higher in fat and sugar content, this country's average life expectancy ranks 30th among more than 100 nations surveyed.

Sadly, within the North American culture, a vast majority of people seem to consider any desire to take naps as a sign of laziness or the behavior of a slothful person who lacks ambition. Within U.S. society we tend to view afternoon naps with suspicion, only seeming to tolerate napping among seniors, the sick or young children.

Understand Basic Napping

Researchers and health professionals at sleep treatment centers have identified three types of basic napping within the U.S. culture:

Habitual: These naps usually occur as a gradually developed habit, generally experienced at the same time daily These shut-eye sessions usually commence right after activities such as exercises like speed-walking, jogging or gym workouts.

Unexpected: Drowsiness sometimes overcomes the individual, occasionally stopping activities such as driving that require the person's full attention.

Planned: Intentionally scheduling naps, such as resting early for events such as a pre-scheduled departure on a lengthy road trip.

Unique Night Shift Challenges

People who work night or "graveyard" shifts report that they sometimes benefit by taking short naps right before the scheduled start of their work shifts.

Especially in instances where such tactics are never used, graveyard workers often experience disruptions in the body's natural circadian rhythm. This biological mechanism serves as the body's internal clock, regulating digestion patterns, the desire and ability to sleep soundly, and various other critical functions.

When the body's natural and usually efficient circadian rhythm gets off kilter, a person might become overly sleepy during work periods. This in turn might decrease the person's job efficiency, while also increasing the probability for accidents.

Some scientists describe these symptoms and the resulting dangers as even worse than "jet lag." That occurs when a person travels to a sharply different time zone. Occasionally jet travel can bump sleep patterns and digestion off kilter, while an unsettled sensation of wooziness become common.

Working in conjunction with physicians, researchers have developed various non-drug treatments often deemed helpful for sluggish night workers and jet lag sufferers.

Some of these people swear to the effectiveness of what many call "light therapy." Those employing this strategy claim that they benefit greatly from the exposure to electric-powered lights much brighter than standard household bulbs.

If true, this means that the lights enable the body to properly adjust its biological clock, particularly if the person is exposed to the bright bulbs several hours before regular wake-up times.

Another treatment method mentioned by the National Sleep Foundation involves taking afternoon naps. But the organization adds this caveat: "Remember that a short (less than 30 minute) nap in the mid to later afternoon may give you energy in the second half of your day, but realize that such a nap can decrease your nighttime sleep need so that it may take you longer to fall asleep or you may sleep for a shorter time."

Night Shift Workers Beware

Various reports indicate that late-night disruptions generated by the exposure to bright lights can sharply disrupt the body's circadian rhythm or internal clock—vastly accelerating the individual's aging process.

So far, significant studies on this specific biological mechanism have only been performed on rats. Yet some scientists indicate that night shift workers have great reason for concern based on these findings, subject to possible change or updates pending any additional research on humans.

In conducting the study reported in the October 2009 issue of "*Aging*," the Russian researchers described basics of the test:

Group: Researchers divided 411 rats including 208 males into four groups.

Environment: Each group was subjected to different levels of light during night hours.

Variances: The separate levels of light ranged from bright light to complete darkness.

Disturbing results: Life spans shortened among the male and female rats that were exposed to natural light and also constant light during the night hours.

For people who are not night workers, this might mean that they should consider taking advantage of daytime light—and perhaps sleep in total darkness if possible at night.

Largely as a result of such findings, some health experts suggest to nightshift workers that they consider finding jobs at other times of the day.

Nightshift workers unable or unwilling to find such employment should strive to ensure that their daytime sleeping environment is kept in total darkness. Taking short but intense "power naps" amid breaks during work also can help reduce disruptions in the body's natural clock.

Unless such measures are taken, some scientists believe,

nightshift workers should expect a shorter lifespan and perhaps a sharp increase in the potential onset of disease.

Benefit from These Extraordinary Nap Tips

Many high-power business executives who often work stressful long days have frequently enhanced their mental performance by often taking "power naps."

Scientists and especially NASA astronauts have long known the benefits of taking brief naps to prevent fatigue, to avoid forgetfulness and to prevent irritability.

Such naps even can "enhance information processing and learning," according to a Harvard University study on napping. Researchers believe that naps clear the mind, opening a pathway for retaining and absorbing critical information.

A primary goal in increasing the efficiency of such naps often involves awakening before the body reverts into the deepest stages of sleep. Those who wait too long, awakening before the deepest sleep begins sometimes complain that upon awakening they feel overly disoriented or groggy.

Napping too long or taking naps late in the day might hamper or worsen any nighttime sleep problems the person already has been experiencing.

Various sleep experts have chronicled numerous reports that recommend taking power naps of no longer than 20 minutes. Napping just 10 minutes longer, at least one half hour or more reportedly can impair a person's physical and mental functions.

Shorter Naps Work Best

Naps of exactly 10 minutes produce the most benefits in reducing sleepiness and enhancing cognitive performance, according to a study reported in the journal "*Sleep*."

The study found that naps in shorter duration and especially much longer naps actually produced less benefit.

Delving deeper in their research, in 2006 scientists strived to compile medical evidence among healthy adults on the potential setbacks and benefits of daytime naps.

As reported in "*Current Opinion Pulmonary Medicine*," afternoon naps restore wakefulness, while also promoting the ability to learn and overall performance.

"Several investigators have shown that napping for as short as 10 minutes improves performance," the article said. "Naps of less than 30 minutes in duration confer several benefits, whereas longer naps are associated with a loss of productivity and sleep inertia. Recent epidemiological studies indicate that frequent and longer naps may lead to adverse long-term health effects."

Particularly during recent years, growing numbers of homeopathic physicians have given their patients such advice, particularly people who complain of afternoon irritability or sluggish mental functions during the daytime.

Pre-scheduled afternoon naps should last about 10 minutes or perhaps 20 minutes at most. Rather than setting alarm clocks, some people have demonstrated a keen ability to train their minds to force themselves to awaken.

At least by some accounts, the mind and more specifically our thought processes can play a significant role in how we individually set our biological clocks. Potential benefits in honing such natural skills enable some people to predictably and easily awaken in the morning at pre-set times such as 6 o'clock.

People unsure of their mental abilities in this realm or who have not yet tested their self-awakening skills should set alarm bells to sound at pre-specified times on clocks, wristwatches or cell phones.

Interest in Naps Intensifies

Overall, the majority of the general public has become increasingly interested in naps during recent years, perhaps due to today's increasingly hectic, fast-paced society.

Add this to the fact that large numbers of people report sleep problems, and the reasons for increasing public interest in the subject becomes increasingly apparent.

Eager to help satisfy public demand for critical and helpful information on such queries, the National Sleep Foundation has developed numerous suggestions.

At the start, people reviewing these tips should understand that the recommendations are not intended to address the needs of individuals suffering from certain severe health issues. Any person within these health-issue categories has unique needs that the following tips are not meant to address.

Right away scientists stress that patients often can easily identify the underlying causes of their own sleep problems. Frequent issues mentioned earlier involving jet lag when changing time zones should seem apparent.

Typically people traveling westbound experience less severe jet lag issues than those going east. Only under the advice and direction of a licensed medical expert or doctor, certain low-dose medications often help eliminate or lessen jet lag issues like grogginess.

One frequent and often-effective remedy for jet lag is melatonin, a naturally occurring substance within the body that helps regulate a person's biological clock. Melatonin plays such a critical and essential role every person's overall health and sleep patterns that Chapter 14 is fully dedicated to this topic.

2
Stay Youthful With REM Sleep

Scientists and doctors generally agree that sleep patterns drastically change among most people after surpassing age 50.

The body's natural and pre-scheduled decrease in production of growth hormones gradually or sometimes rapidly accelerates signs of aging the sleep quality and times of a person gradually degrade.

Considered by many doctors and lay people as a vicious cycle, this predictable and expected biological development is especially vile in the eyes of many older people.

As the years steadily click past the vast majority of older people experience the wreckage of sound-sleep, the obliteration of a pattern that they once enjoyed and benefited markedly from.

For these people natural sleep patterns become a mere sweet memory, predictable, lengthy and deep resting cycles once prevalent through childhood, youth, young adult years and middle age.

For most seniors the loss of sleep generates a pattern that remains through the remainder of their lives. These unwanted developments include the onset of wrinkles, hair loss, a decrease in cognitive ability, gradual failure of the body's vital organs and eventually death.

As mentioned earlier, devising and maintaining effective ways of regaining effective, healthy sleep patterns can go a long way toward slowing, stalling or even halting at least some of these many developments that many people label as "negative."

Compounding matters, when a senior citizen develops various new health problems these afflictions often leads to the onset of additional sleep issues. These combined patterns can lead to a "cascading effect," rapidly accelerating advanced signs of aging and quickly resulting in death.

The Elixir of Life

For good reason the growth hormones naturally produced within our bodies have been hailed as the "elixir of life." All this becomes possible thanks to your body's critical rapid-eye movement or REM sleep.

During that sleep stage the pituitary gland pumps out large quantities of HGH, a precursor to the IGF-1 produced in the liver. From the pituitary gland the blood carries the HGH to the liver, which transforms that crucial substance into essential IGF-1—the working molecule of HGH.

Since infancy the growth hormone enables us to retain our youthful qualities, grow steadily through childhood through the teen years, develop and maintain critical muscle mass and even to heal from serious wounds or fight disease.

Simply stated, without REM you would not have human growth hormone which is essential and critically necessary for every human being to remain alive.

Naturally, the body's production of natural internal HGH steadily wanes as people mature, generating the often-unwanted qualities of aging among seniors.

All animals suffer negative health impacts when continually or repeatedly awakened from sleep, particularly REM.

In one study sleep-deprived rats lived only an average of five weeks when deprived of REM, compared to the normal three-year lifespan of that species. Disturbingly, the tails and paws of the sleep-deprived rats emitted a signal of apparent immune system problems in those regions, the lowering of temperatures.

For anyone concerned with sleep issues, such results become even more shocking when realizing that humans deprived of sleep suffer even more negative health issues.

According to published reports, scientists lacked any inkling that the REM sleep process existed until 1953. Intense testing since then has proven inconclusively that the body produces the bulk of growth hormone for brief spans of less than 30 minutes during brief periods of rapid-eye sleep before gradually diminishing.

Break this Vicious Cycle

According to a vast array of medical literature, some researchers contend that regaining or increasing critical rapid-eye or REM sleep can slow or stall aging.

REM is an essential phase of sleep during which the body generates the critical human growth hormone commonly called "HGH," essential in generating youthful attributes. REM reigns as essential to life among all mammals in order to maintain vitality, youthfulness and vigor, plus overall physical health and mental acuity.

Increasingly mindful of these factors, I'm among homeopaths who contend that boosting REM sleep among seniors can help markedly increase their youthfulness.

Well documented research confirms that infants spend half of their sleep time in REM sleep. That compares to just 20 percent of sleep time among young and middle-aged adults. These levels drop off even more among seniors.

Essential Sleep Stages

Before striving to rejuvenate the amount and quality of their REM sleep, seniors should first understand the characteristics that people undergo amid such rest.

Perhaps most notably, amid rapid-eye sleep a person's breathing usually becomes irregular, quicker and shallow. Wide-awake people observing an individual amid REM notice that the sleeper's eyes seem to jerk rapidly in various directions.

While the arms and legs become temporarily paralyzed amid this state, blood pressures and heart rates increase.

Any attempts to awaken people experiencing REM are far more difficult than striving to arouse someone undergoing lower-stage "light sleep." Anyone awakened amid deep-stage REM sleep often vividly remembers dreams from when the moment that he or she is aroused.

Many of the most intense, healthful dreams occur during the REM stage, which usually occurs for the first time each night on average around 90 minutes after bedtime.

According to the National Sleep Foundation this initial REM state, usually lasting 10 minutes or less, marks the person's first of numerous rapid-eye stages for the night.

Particularly among people whose sleep goes undisturbed, throughout the wee hours of the morning subsequent REM episodes steadily increase in depth and in length.

Although some people immediately forget or have no recall of their dreams, for lots of us the best recall of dreaming happens briefly upon awakening in the morning.

All these compelling details essentially add up to the fact that our aging process is likely to slow if and when we successfully experience full nights of undisturbed sleep—generating more REM and thereby enabling the body to increase its growth hormone production.

Avoid Distracting Saboteurs

Necessary to achieve any hope of anti-aging sleep, every adult and particularly seniors needs to avoid certain food, drinks or lifestyle habits that can disturb REM.

Besides caffeinated drinks, decongestants and diet pills, some of the worst disruptors triggering insomnia or sleep issues include smoking, alcohol and extreme temperatures—either too hot or too cold. These various disruptions disturb sleep and particularly REM.

Also potentially poking a proverbial dagger into any good-sleep efforts designed to maximize REM, antidepressants disturb neurotransmitters within the brain—disrupting or blocking rapid-eye movement.

Numerous Issues Emerge

A vast array studies clearly indicate that REM generates substantial benefits to young people, particularly infants and children when this crucial brain activity stimulates the brain's ability to learn.

Additional research has indicated that adults who have

recently been taught a new skill tend to lose such memory when deprived of REM.

Robbing people of this natural activity also can wreak havoc on daytime moods, decreasing optimism regarding life. Such mental prophesies essential evolve into self-fulfilling life plans among many people who suffer the extensive loss of REM.

Many scientists generally believe such people are less inclined to take the risks, lifestyle choices that can open pathways for substantial life achievements.

Read This Vital Summary

By understanding, learning and appreciating the many topics, lessons and suggestions that follow, you'll have the basic tools necessary to effectively and naturally increase and experience the wondrous anti-aging sleep that REM helps provide.

3
Hidden Challenges Rob You of Quality Sleep

The late U.S. novelist F. Scott Fitzgerald once famously wrote, "It appears that every man's insomnia is as different from his neighbor's as are their daytime hopes and aspirations."

At some point in their lives at least 58 percent of Americans are afflicted by sleep disorders including insomnia.

Scientists and medical professionals cite a vast list of reasons.

At the start, sleep experts often suggest that patients complaining of sleep issues ask themselves a handful of basic questions. Among the most basic queries that many doctors want their patients to ponder. Doctors say that those answering "yes" to any of these questions might be suffering from one or more potentially unhealthful sleep issues:

Performance: Does your mind lose its sharpness, particularly toward the end of the work day?

Mental acuity: Does your mind lose an ability to focus on a particular subject, particularly after you have sat in one place for a lengthy period?

Triggers: Does your body and mind fail to reach peak efficiency unless a stimulant such as coffee is taken?

Moodiness: Does your mood evolve into gloomy tones as the day progresses?

Pitfalls of Self-Diagnosis

As a physician I always strongly urge consumers to avoid making any attempt to diagnose their own physical conditions. Only a medical professional should do that.

Even so, before visiting a doctor many people want to know if they likely suffer from insomnia, which can emerge as a serious medical condition.

When patients complaining of sleep problems visit my clinic, I tell them that many of their individual lifestyle choices or habits might be hindering or blocking the body's natural mechanisms that normally generate sleepiness. The most frequent culprits here are often energy drinks, coffee and other stimulants.

While the specific causes of insomnia vary, many patients suffering from this condition often realize or sense that their performance or alertness has deteriorated.

Such occurrences often generate issues or challenges in personal safety and with the overall welfare of the general public as well. Examples of such instances sometimes involve overly sleepy people who foolishly, recklessly or unknowingly attempt to drive

Just as important, at least from an overall perspective insomnia can indirectly generate adverse impacts on a person's family life and relationships. Additionally, an impaired ability to make sound judgments can trigger negative life-changing events, including potentially extreme difficulties in the work environment.

Doctor Helene A. Emsellem, medical director of The Center for Sleep & Wake Disorders, defines insomnia this way: "If you feel that you're getting an insufficient amount of sleep and it's happening on a regular basis, then we consider that to be insomnia.

If you're having difficulty falling asleep or staying asleep—some individuals may fall asleep fine but wake up between two and five in the morning and not be able to sleep the final portion of the night. Any of these patterns may be considered insomnia."

With these factors and potential dangers clearly understood, people diagnosed with insomnia or at the very least some other form of mysterious chronic sleep loss—or who worry they suffer from such conditions—first need to clearly identify a specific cause. So whether you're aware of being sleep deprived, or you're just in denial about your condition, the obvious question to ask is "why?"

You'll need clear and concise answers to such queries before being able to take decisive and effective action to eliminate or minimize the problem.

Review and Consider the Potential Physical Maladies

Through hundreds of years of intense research on the issue, particularly within the past few decades, scientists have identified specific medical conditions that often rob the body of its alertness levels or of the vital need to meet minimum sleep requirements.

Some of the most prevalent culprits are potentially debilitating medical conditions including sleep apnea, diabetes and thyroid dysfunction. Only physicians can effectively treat such problems.

Additional causes often can be handled by patients who modify their lifestyle habits or daily food and beverage choices.

The following are some of the most common triggers of sleep disorders, which patients can review to start pondering the likely causes of their own conditions.

Restless Legs Syndrome: Contrary to some "urban legends," this condition never involves sleep walking.

Instead, this entails a serious medical condition where the legs move or jerk as a direct result of a neurological movement disorder within the body's nervous system.

"Doctor, I have a strange prickling or tingling feeling in my legs," many patients suffering from this syndrome say when interacting with their doctors.

Senior citizens are the most likely segment of the population to begin suffering from this condition, although the syndrome can strike people at any age.

Diabetes has been listed among the most frequent triggering factors that potentially ignite sleep issues.

Whatever the underlying cause, restless legs syndrome often fragments or hampers the person's ability to get necessary sleep, thereby generating chronic insomnia. Many patients suffering from this disorder complain of being repeatedly awakened at any time of day.

Researchers have estimated that at least one out of every ten people in North America and Europe suffer from at least some degree of restless legs syndrome—particularly individuals in the latter stages of a normal life span.

To control, manage or minimize the symptoms, doctors usually strive to manage levels of a natural neurotransmitter within the body—dopamine. Physicians usually select from among various drugs in attempts to handle this chore.

Sleep Apnea: Those most prone to this extremely dangerous condition primarily are people over age 50. As compared to the general population many people with this condition have greater body fat buildup.

Sleep apnea can impact any age group, but seniors are more prone to develop the condition. The danger intensifies when a loss in muscle tone and the buildup of fats around the throat occasionally collapses the upper pharynx amid sleep.

Scientists call the most dangerous levels of this condition "obstructive sleep apnea." Worse-case scenarios can cause death while sleeping, or even severe disorders within the brain or other vital organs due to a lack of oxygen for extended periods.

By some accounts, sleep apnea afflicts at least 18 million Americans. The problem is so widespread that the overall danger throughout society might be far worse than generally believed by most people.

The critical nature of the overall situation comes into clear focus when considering the fact that only a handful of people suffering from sleep apnea have been diagnosed as having the condition.

This disease or disorder is often associated with snoring. Yet some people with the condition do not snore at all.

The danger comes into clear focus to people with sleep apnea and their relatives upon learning that the condition occasionally blocks air flow for as many as 10 seconds.

People inside the same room as a person suffering from sleep apnea often become concerned when they hear the person's snoring intermittently stops for extended periods.

Oxygen levels fall in the blood, essentially putting the individual in critical danger. Some suffers invariably awaken at least momentarily, a symptom that occasionally results in insomnia.

The problem becomes increasingly critical, pushing up the chances for various diseases including stroke, memory loss, depression, cardiovascular disease and congestive heart failure. Respiratory arrest due to windpipe closure amid sleep sometimes causes sudden death.

The overall danger often worsens due to the fact that such episodes sometimes occur literally hundreds of times in a single night among some individuals with sleep apnea.

While sleeping many sleep apnea sufferers snort or gasp as their bodies instinctively strive to re-open the windpipe. Much of the time, particularly among people unaware that they suffer from sleep apnea, the person awakens in the mornings feeling extremely sleepy.

Understandably, the National Sleep Foundation recommends that physicians who diagnose the condition immediately begin treatments in order to prevent or minimize the probability of serious diseases worsening

Especially among patients who remain untreated, complaints of serious morning headaches are quite prevalent. Also, besides an occasional loss in mental clarity, some sleep apnea sufferers become irritable or lose interest in physical intimacy.

Well aware of this condition's potentially severe problems, I sometimes tell patients that "if you can hear the sleeping person snoring or breathing from another room, that could be a significant warning sign of potential sleep apnea."

The degree of concern should increase if the sleeping person is heard gasping, stops breathing, makes loud noises or gasps.

Children suffering from sleep apnea occasionally suffer from a variety of unique ailments that do not usually impact senior citizens who have the affliction.

Rapid and heavy breathing often emerge as among symptoms in children with sleep apnea. Key factors triggering this disorder in children include obesity, and Attention Deficit Hyperactivity Disorder. This sometimes disturbs a child's sleep.

Get Vital Medical Tests

Specialized sleep centers have unique technology enabling the facilities to conduct polysomnography tests. These examinations enable physicians or highly trained medical professionals to analyze various bodily functions, particularly brain waves.

Physicians often use the results to determine if a patient has sleep apnea. Doctors employ various treatment methods, geared to each patient's needs, symptoms and the likely cause of that individual's sleep disorder. Overall severity levels and treatments often recommended within those categories include:

Mild: Many doctors help launch weight-loss regimens, while administering treatments designed to help patients adjust their bodily positions while sleeping. Lots of physicians believe that sleeping on both sides or on the stomach can help minimize or eliminate windpipe closure.

Severe: Surgery sometimes becomes necessary to clear obstructions within the body's upper airways. Mask-like devices called C-PAP machines are often used, even in instances where operations are not required or recommended.

Unique treatments: At least one test as reported by the British Medical Journal has concluded that playing the Didgeridoo—an indigenous Australian Aborigine musical wind instrument—has been an "effective treatment." The study's 25 participants played such instruments at least five days per week, about 25 minutes per session. Following at least four months of such routines, the study said that most participants experienced "profound improvement" in their apnea conditions.

Beware of Non-prescribed Pills

People suffering from sleep apnea must always remain fully cognizant of the fact that pills should never be considered as a "cure-all." This should be a continual mental mantra among all such patients, particularly those whose doctors never prescribed drugs.

Most important in this regard, I'm among physicians who strongly warn sleep apnea patients to avoid taking sleeping pills or various other sedatives.

The danger emerges or intensifies when such medications prevent people with sleep apnea from reawakening, a natural physical response that would enable the individual to resume breathing. Remember, unless the windpipe opens serious organ damage or death can occur.

Various Bodily Functions

A wide variety of physical ailments, diseases and conditions can adversely impact sleep. When this happens overall health becomes endangered. The most prevalent physical conditions include diabetes mellitus, asthma, immune system disorders and gastroesophageal reflux disease.

The basic types of sleep disorders or problems impacting or caused by some of these conditions include:

Narcolepsy: People with this hereditary condition

intermittently suffer unexpected spells of sleep or "sleep attacks." The condition often robs the person of vital nighttime sleep. Danger intensifies when sudden, unexpected and spontaneous daytime sleep episodes last up to 30 minutes. Researchers blame a serious disorder that disables genes that otherwise would regulate brain cell functions within healthy people. When working correctly, these brain cells effectively communicate with other cells throughout the body. Some doctors prefer to prescribe various medications in order to manage, minimize or eliminate the dangerous sudden sleep episodes. Other research indicates that scheduling and taking daytime naps at pre-set times might serve as an effective natural antidote.

Sleep Problems Sometimes Afflict Women

A wide variety of research reports over the past several generations indicate that women sometimes suffer from unique sleep problems that men rarely if ever experience. The National Sleep Foundation reports a number of gender-specific sleep issues impacting women. Among findings that pinpoint differences in how the genders sleep, primarily triggered by females experiencing menopause, pregnancy and menstrual cycles:

(*) As an overall sector of the general population, women get sleepier during the daytime, experience difficulty staying asleep at night and have more difficulty falling asleep at bedtime as compared to men, according to a 2005 survey.

(*) The average nightly sleep periods on weeknights are only six hours and 41 minutes among U.S. women ages 30 to 60.

The various biological cycles start and end in phases during a woman's life. Some of the most significant changes click on and off as the hormones progesterone and estrogen play varying roles in the natural cycles of women's bodies.

These various transitions last from the teens well into the advanced senior years. Adding to this challenge, women often experience sleep disruptions caused by a variety of environmental factors. Perhaps noise or other disturbances such as crying babies, howling winds or extremely inclement weather bothers women more than men.

Appreciate, Recognize and Treat Gender Differences

Many sleep experts urge women to consider a variety of natural, non-invasive and non-pharmaceutical methods to increase the duration and quality of their sleep.

Among some of the most prevalent suggestions in this regard:

Exercise: Adding a workout regimen that's not too strenuous but rigorous enough to change the body's patterns often generates sleepiness and more restful sleep.

Diet: Eliminating naturally stimulating foods such as caffeine often helps the body gradually revert back to more natural and restful sleep patterns.

Schedule: Forming and sticking to pre-set sleep and awake-times can help the body revert to a healthful, predictable pattern.

Various studies as reported by the Sleep Foundation have indicated positive results among people adopting some or all of these basic changes.

One study showed a marked improvement in the sleep patterns of post-menopausal obese women who began morning exercise. As an overall group, women who participated in this study gradually started sleeping more soundly and longer. Related research found that women who exercised in the mornings benefited more than those who exercised primarily during the evenings.

Pain Interrupts Women's Sleep

Pain from injuries or various physical ailments is more likely to prevent or hamper the sleep of women as opposed to men, according to a Sleep Foundation survey.

A full 58 percent of women surveyed complained that for periods lasting more than one week pain had interrupted their sleep at least three nights per week. Only 48 percent of men reported similar problems.

Women suffered specific types of pain frequently associated with disrupting or preventing sleep.

Besides migraines, the most common pain-causing conditions most likely to afflict women than men include heartburn, tension headaches, rheumatic disorders and arthritis.

Rather than rely on dangerous or potentially addictive drugs to manage the pain, many homeopaths and sleep experts recommend a variety of non-pharmaceutical remedies. Depending on the individual's specific conditions, these strategies can include cognitive therapy biofeedback, and relaxation techniques.

4
Warning:
All Snoring is Unhealthy

Although almost all societies consider snoring as "natural," virtually every instance of this condition should actually be considered unhealthy, many sleep experts say.

Such a revelation might initially seem shocking or unbelievable. After all, virtually all of us either snores at least somewhat or knows someone who does on a regular basis.

Certainly the mere fact that a person snores does not necessarily signify an extremely serious medical condition. Yet some sleep experts and doctors suggest that you should always be on the lookout for potentially important warning signs, such as:

Strange sounds: Traumatic huffing, puffing and wheezing, especially sounds that seem unusual or what a common observer might call "unusual or unnatural snoring."

Annoyance: You should become concerned if you hear snoring that annoys you, or if someone tells you that they feel irritated by the sound of your snoring.

Disruptions: An additional reason for concern should erupt if you're occasionally or frequently awakened by the sound of your own snoring, or if a loved one experiences this.

Chronic: Mental alarm bells should sound if such irritating episodes of snoring continue on a fairly regular or nightly basis.

"This is a potentially serious matter, not a reason for making jokes," I tell patients who report such experiences.

Patients need to understand that extreme episodes of snoring are common, far from unusual. Various research reports have indicated that at least 30 percent of women and 45 percent of men are chronic snorers.

Consider Celebrities Who Died

My various other articles and books through the years, including the "Healing Power of Sleep," have noted that numerous celebrities or world figures have died at least in part due to sleep problems that in some instances exacerbated their snoring. Among them:

Queen Victoria of Britain: Her snoring worsened as her weight increased with age, dying of a stroke in 1901 at age 81.

President Theodore Roosevelt: Suffered from chronic snoring, dying from a coronary embolism while sleeping at age 60 in 1919.

President Franklin Delano Roosevelt: Suffered from a severe case of sleep apnea before dying in his sleep at age 63 in 1945.

Of course, the vast majority of chronic snorers who die as a direct or partial result of sleep disorders are everyday people rather than celebrities. Even so, mentioning the names of just a handful of widely known individuals who died while suffering from sleep disorders helps put the overall health issue into perspective.

Understand the Basics of Snoring

In almost all species of mammals including humans snoring occurs when the natural air flow gets disrupted or obstructed.

Besides the increase in bodily fats associated with older age as mentioned earlier, some of the most common causes include muscle tension within misaligned jaws, sudden or extensive bodily weight gain, weakened throat muscles and nasal passage obstructions.

Scientists insist that snoring occurs most frequently during a person's deepest stages of sleep. This phase is commonly called rapid-eye movement or REM sleep.

When within this stage, the eyes move extremely rapidly— almost always behind the closed eyelids. If you observe a sleeping person whose eyelids appear to twitch, this might indicate that the individual is in the process of experiencing REM sleep.

While all this might seem rather strange or odd to casual observers, the REM process is actually essential to human life and to good health. This is largely because during REM the pituitary gland within the brain secretes vital hormones that help regulate various organ functions and help keep you alive.

Perhaps the most essential of these naturally occurring substances are "human growth hormones," sometimes called HGH.

During childhood, adolescence and our young adult years, HGH enables the body's organs to grow at a healthy and pre-scheduled predictable rate—while also helping to naturally strengthen the muscles.

Critical Period for Snoring

The frequency of chronic or severe snoring during REM sleep intensifies danger to the person's overall health. Sudden death thus becomes a possibility during intense rapid-eye movement sleep, particularly if the snoring person has sleep apnea.

Added danger comes to both young and senior people who snore often. Among dangers:

Children: Chronic snorers might suffer growth or organ problems, since snoring or related sleep disorders might hinder the body's maturation processes.

Young adults: Particularly due to the production of HGH during deep sleep, sound and steady rest is essential to heal from wounds and to prevent diseases.

Middle age: Chronic snorers within this age bracket might experience a deterioration of overall health, potentially a "domino effect" where organ functions steadily worsen.

Seniors: Largely due to the suppression of HGH, chronic snoring could hinder recovery from various ailments or weaken the body's ability to prevent diseases.

The potential dangers sometimes increase among all age groups of snorers during REM sleep when the body sends natural messages for all muscles in the body to relax.

Critical organs and structures in the body's breathing mechanisms naturally relax, including the palate, tongue and throat. Sudden or severe health problems or even death might occur in some instances where sleep apnea shuts down the windpipe, when breathing structures are far too relaxed to respond in time to awaken the person.

Chronic Snoring Dangers Abound

To varying degrees and depending on individual circumstances, the challenges facing chronic snorers often are similar to those afflicting people with sleep apnea.

Besides potential depression, people who suffer snoring

problems sometimes suffer from a wide range of issues that include a loss of sex drive and increased irritability.

Sadly, rather than striving to address the underlying health issues that cause their snoring, some people simply buy earplugs while striving to avoid the issue.

"Avoid falling into a trap that has eventually harmed many innocent, well-intended people," I occasionally tell patients. "Far too many people make the critical mistake of incorrectly believing that chronic snoring is a harmless or benign condition."

From my experience now in my fifth decade of medical practice, far too many people mistakenly believe that snoring is merely a harmless byproduct of aging.

Thankfully, numerous physicians and good-health consultants have steadily and frequently maintained an effort to inform the public about the dangers of snoring.

Among the strongest leaders here has been Doctor Sanjay Gupta, a resident medical authority at the CNN-TV cable television news network. Among Gupta's many essential warnings about sleep issues, as mentioned in his column on CNN's Website:

Warning sign: Chronic or loud snoring can be a warning sign that the person might have the more serious overall condition of sleep apnea. This in turn also increases the probability that the individual might suffer from a variety of health issues often connected with that ailment, such as diabetes, hypertension and heart disease.

Stroke factors: Within the neck's arteries partly as an apparent result of excessive snoring, plaque buildup emerges as a major risk factor for stroke. Shockingly, a leading medical study indicates that snoring increases 10-fold the likelihood of atherosclerosis that generates the neck's plaque build-up.

Alcohol: The nightly consumption of alcohol right before bedtime can sharply increase chances that the person will snore all night. This, in turn, increases the probability that the individual will develop sleep apnea.

Actively Treat Chronic Snoring

Everyone who snores often or loudly should immediately take decisive action to eliminate the problem, because otherwise serious health issues are likely to develop—if such conditions have not already emerged.

Perhaps just as important, patients who snore need to know that treating that condition might decrease, eliminate or lesson other debilitating conditions that they suffer from. Migraines and daytime irritability are among symptoms that sometimes decrease or disappear when treatments or lifestyle changes end a person's snoring.

Behavioral Changes Become Preferable

Just like in most sleep apnea cases, with snoring a modification in behavior sometimes emerges effective. This is far more preferable than using overly expensive and often-ineffective drugs, some potentially harmful that might give questionable results.

Among the behavior changes that many sleep experts and doctors recommend for snorers, depending on each patient's individual circumstances:

Quit Smoking: Tobacco use at any level sharply increases the likelihood of many diseases including cancer and heart disease.

The early or later stages of smoking, even at minimal levels, can trigger snoring that generates a negative "cascading effect." Smoking often irritates the throat, windpipe and lungs, thereby causing a person to snore.

Weight loss: Amid people of all ages, excessive body fat sometimes exacerbates or even ignites snoring. Some studies suggest that the propensity for a particular individual to snore decreases markedly for every 10 pounds lost.

Sleeping position: Avoid sleeping on your back, because doing so often naturally blocks the body's natural airways. Sleeping on the back sharply increases the probability of chronic snoring. Instead, you should strive to sleep on your stomach or sides through the entire night. Various studies have shown that this single modification can often go a long way toward eliminating or decreasing snoring in many individuals.

Many people who prefer to sleep alone, lacking a bed partner who might encourage them to sleep in certain positions, have developed a clever way to stay off their backs. This clever strategy involves fastening small or mid-size, relatively harmless golf balls to the back-side of pajama tops or T-shirts that are worn while sleeping. The uncomfortable protrusion invariably forces the person to sleep on his or her stomach or sides.

The strategy often works among patients who have generally slept on their backs for their entire lives. Other help also sometimes comes from loving, compassionate or understanding bed partners who encourage snorers to roll off their backs.

Avoidance: Another key strategy often entails avoiding alcohol or drugs, particularly before bedtime. Remember, those substances sometimes relax or loosen the body's breathing structures; increasing the probability the person will develop chronic snoring. In many instances, some doctors and sleep experts say, people who stop drinking or taking medications before bedtime immediately or gradually lose the propensity to snore.

Severe Cases Involve More Aggressive Treatments

More aggressive treatment regimens often become necessary in cases of severe snoring cases where weight loss, smoking cessation, and drug avoidance and sleep position changes have failed.

Rather than merely going to a standard physician, at this point some patients might want to consider going to a professional sleep study and treatment center. Such facilities specialize in diagnosing and specific treatments for a wide variety of sleep disorders.

For the most part, surgery is often considered a less desirable option. Nonetheless, blockages in the body sometimes motivate doctors to urge patients to take such action.

In addition, for certain instances doctors recommend using specialized steroids in order to reduce bodily symptoms that can lead to snoring. Such conditions usually involve obstructions or hindrances such as inflamed nasal passages or swollen throats.

Although steroids often generate temporary or short-term relief from conditions that trigger or exacerbate snoring, such medications usually involve health risks.

Medical Devices Often Become Preferable

A wide variety of medical devices including specialized surgical implants for certain cases often become a treatment option before drug or after lifestyle-change efforts fail.

Dental mouthpieces: These devices usually strive to keep the jaw or the body's other internal breathing mechanisms into certain positions. The goal is to keep the airways open to prevent or decrease any interruptions in breathing. Holding the jaw forward often becomes a primary goal, using form-fitting dental devices sized and created to meet the individual patient's mouth structure and bone alignment needs. This often proves effective. However, physicians warn of potential dangers including jaw pain, dry mouths, facial discomfort, or excessive saliva.

Palatial implants: Physicians or medical professionals inject a polyester filament into the soft palate to stiffen the tissue by creating scar tissue. Doctors sometimes attempt this strategy after mouthpieces have proven ineffective in the individual. Medical professionals usually only consider this strategy after attempts with dental mouthpieces fail. Also, problems with the person's soft palate first must been deemed the cause of snoring.

Continuous positive airway pressure: Doctors consider this option for severe snorers, particularly people with obstructive sleep apnea. Worn over the nose while sleeping, this pressurized mask is connected to a small pump that maintains high air pressure. Ideally this prevents sleep apnea and snoring by keeping the body's airways open. Yet potential problems sometimes erupt. Some patients complain of discomfort when wearing the masks all night. Noise from the machine also sometimes disturbs the patients or their bed partners.

Final Option: Surgical Procedures

Some physicians offer surgical procedures as a potential final option, only after medical devices, lifestyle changes or drugs have failed.

Unlike during much of the late 20th Century, many of today's surgeries to eliminate snoring are considered non-invasive. Any potential need to cut body tissue with a knife is often unnecessary, thanks to various new devices and updated procedures.

Among today's most frequent surgical techniques, many considered far less painful as operations performed as recently as the 1990s:

Lasers: Doctors strengthen the soft palate or remove obstructions from airways. Most surgeries are done on an "out-patient basis." The surgery is performed at the physician's office, which the patient leaves on the same day as the procedure. The surgeon uses a small hand-held beam to prevent the palate from excessively vibrating, thereby lessening or eliminating any snoring. Sleep apnea patients usually are not considered candidates for this procedure, which usually requires multiple surgical procedures performed on different days.

Radiofrequency tissue ablation: Rather than attempt to strengthen the soft palate in an attempt to lessen or eliminate snoring, the doctor removes part of the organ with a low-intensity radio frequency signal. This procedure opens the nasal passageways. The operation is performed on an out-patient basis, usually within 15 minutes. The doctor and patient need three months to determine if the procedure has been a success. Two out of three patients who undergo this surgery consider the procedure as successful in decreasing or eliminating their snoring. Yet some research indicates a high relapse rate.

Traditional surgery: After other procedures fail this procedure under general anesthesia in a hospital operating room is usually considered only as a last resort. Such procedures often involve a deviated septum, usually a crooked or loose defect in the border between the nostrils. Some individuals have a deviated septum at birth. Allergies also sometimes cause potential problems in the nasal passages, gradually generating polyps of mucus growth.

5

Consult Medical Professionals

The importance of relying on a doctor or licensed medical professional in diagnosing, identifying and treating sleep issues should remain an essential strategy.

To do otherwise is to invite potential disaster, largely because you might have serious or steadily worsening underlying health issues that need treatment.

Patients who visit physicians for these issues, and even those who avoid doctors, often pinpoint sleeping issues and effective treatments in a trial-and-error process.

Whether under the care of a doctor or on their own, consumers can use some or all of the following National Sleep Foundation suggestions—as long as they're not children or adults with pre-existing health issues.

Examination: For those willing and sensible enough to visit a doctor at the onset of any sleep-improvement effort should, get a thorough medical checkup. This might identify underlying health issues, potential triggers that might cause sleep issues.

Lifestyle decisions: Make sensible choices regarding sleep, such as going to bed at night and awakening at about the same times daily. Doing so might tend to maximize the body's production of human growth hormone or HGH, the naturally occurring substance essential for optimal health at any age.

Predictable Sleep Patterns: One of the most essential tasks entails starting and keeping predictable sleep schedules. Conversely, by continually changing sleep times such as often staying up until 3 o'clock in the morning, while going to bed at 10 at night other days can seriously disrupt the body's natural sleep clock.

Just as important, deciding several mornings weekly to sleep until 10, while getting up at 7 most days, also might play a significant role in disrupting the body's schedule.

Ultimately, living life in such a haphazard fashion could put your digestion and toxic-elimination system off kilter.

Such a situation could lead to organ damage, while weakening immunity and thereby making the body more susceptible to communicable diseases. When the liver, kidneys and other vital organs stop working at peak efficiencies, toxins sometimes build within the body as immunity weakens.

Take Charge of Your Sleep Environment

Besides potentially accelerating the aging process, the bodies of people who wreak havoc on their own bodies' time clocks might become more susceptible to diseases including cancer.

So, whatever age group you are in, be sure to set and maintain a fairly predictable sleep schedule. Rather than taking drugs to induce sleepiness, those who have trouble falling asleep at night should consider daily exposure to at least one hour of morning sunlight.

Pre-Bedtime antics: Avoid arousing activities right before the regular nightly start of sleep time. Never vigorously exercise right before bed, run non-stop errands during such a period or other physically rigorous activities.

Instead, strive to gradually and steadily relax, preferably during the 90 minutes to two hours right before bedtime. This enables the body to revert into the restful mode.

Doing otherwise invites restlessness immediately before and immediately after going to bed. The bodies of most people become energetic and generally stay rigorous for a period of time immediately after intense exercise.

Avoid rough-housing with your children in games like wrestling in the mid-evening or late-night hours. Also, avoid bright lights that might tend to stimulate the brain's neurons, tricking the body into believing that the late evening is the middle of the day.

The only exception to this strategy is sex between consenting adults, usually in the same bed where sleep is planned. As many of us already know, Mother Nature often puts people of both genders into a restful mode after orgasm, particularly men.

Control thought patterns: Worrisome lifestyle issues such as financial problems sometimes keep people awake far longer than intended, long after they've gone to bed.

If such mental anguish hampers your ability to sleep, develop creative ways to "vent" the issue or express your feelings on the matter well before bedtime.

Frequent tactics in this regard include verbalizing the issues when you're alone, speaking calmly about the problem with a trusted friend or relative, or even keeping a daily diary or journal where you write down your private thoughts. All this should be done at least 90 minutes before scheduled bedtime.

Optimally, these tactics will help ease the mind at least

somewhat, increasing the probability of falling asleep with relative ease at the scheduled bedtime.

Bed activities: Adults need to restrict their in-bed activities to two things—sleep or consensual sex.

Engaging in other activities while in bed might seem comfortable. But doing so tends to disrupt or hamper the overall quality and duration of sleep. Competing daily chores like making shopping lists or elective activities such as surfing the Internet are best done outside of bed, sleep experts say.

Remember, sex is okay and even recommended in bed because intimate physical relations often release hormones that induce long, deep sleep.

By performing activities other than sleep and sex while in bed, we invariably teach the mind that such locations are ideal for a variety of activities including excessive worrying. Yet doing so undermines sleep quality, also hampering the ability to fall asleep.

Cozy environment: Trying to sleep in an extremely bright room with the radio blaring obviously is a far-from-optimal condition for rest—at least for most people.

Whether or not we realize this, many of us sleep in bedrooms or areas of our residences that are not conducive or ideal for sleep.

An open door that lets light beam into a room can be just as much of a hindrance as a closed window that prevents essential oxygen from entering the room.

Strangely, many people fail to realize that they often or usually sleep in environments that are far from ideal. Flickering lights and pesky noise from a television watched by a spouse or loved one in the same room might bother sleep patterns and the essential dreaming process, whether or not we realize this is happening.

Some of the biggest offenders are laptop screens, iPad monitors near the eyes of a sleeper. Scientists warn that those glaring devices are on the blue end of the light spectrum, a level considered disruptive to the body's natural inner clock.

The varying potentially distracting things can often be effectively eliminated or minimized at little or no cost. Low-cost measures can include buying en eye mask to block tiny beams of light, covering the display on a digital bedside clock, and wearing inexpensive earplugs to block or minimize noise.

Some consumers use clever ways to effectively mask or minimize bothersome noise such as the sounds of traffic from nearby streets or jet aircraft far overhead in neighborhoods close to airports.

The secret involves generating "white noise." This strategy usually involves using such devices as high-power fans that create a non-bothersome continual whooshing noise, or using radios, DVDs and computers. Some insomniacs continuously play soothing sounds such as waterfalls, gurgling mountain streams or waves gently cascading repetitively across a beach.

Another equally important tactic, although usually much more expensive, usually entails buying new and far more comfortable furniture and bedroom accessories. A cozy pillow and a comfortable bed can go a long way toward promoting restful sleep.

Also, remove dust or potential allergens that bother many

people. One of the most important tactics involves maintaining an optimal sleep temperature.

Sleep Positions: As mentioned earlier, sleep positions often play an essential role in whether a person is likely to snore. Consumers also need to know that the position a person rests in can profoundly impact sleep quality.

Particularly among patients older than 49, I give a variety of suggestions on sleep positions. The sleep positions recommended for each patient usually hinge on the individual's specific health issues.

Certain positions tend to disrupt sleep or potentially exacerbate pre-existing negative health conditions. My basic recommendations include:

Left side: People suffering from gastroesophageal disease or stomach reflex issues usually do better when sleeping on this side of the body. Other frequent candidates for this sleep position include people with left-lung fluid buildup, emphysema, and snoring problems. When people sleep on their left sides, the efficiency usually increases within the three-lobed right lung, as opposed to the two-lobed left lung.

Right side: People suffering from what doctors call "flabby hearts" or the buildup of fluids in the right lungs usually benefit from sleeping on this side of the body.

The back: As stated earlier, among chronic snorers the back usually is by far the least preferable side of the body to sleep on. Sleeping on the left side is preferable for most of them.

Arm and hand: The positions of these limbs and extremities can become a nuisance during sleep, particularly when placed under the head.

Besides interrupting or hampering sleep, excessively or even occasionally sleeping in this position can result in neck problems, headaches, circulatory problems or numbness in the hands or limbs. People suffering from circulation problems, arthritis or carpel tunnel syndrome should strive to avoid this sleep position.

Stomach: At least most of the time, this position generally seems to have little or no adverse impact on sleep quality or overall health.

Other Helpful Tips Emerge

Thanks to increasingly intensive research on various sleep issues, scientists have developed additional tips designed to maximize sleep quality while eliminating substances and lifestyle habits that curtail that activity. Among them:

Food and beverages: People suffering from various sleep issues ranging from insomnia to sleep apnea need to always remain cognizant of foods they eat.

Consuming large meals or drinking excessive alcohol sometimes tends to put people into deep REM sleep or prevent any rest. Research shows that eating big meals sometimes puts the digestive track into overdrive, causing so much stimulation within the body that sleep becomes difficult.

Drinking too many beverages can cause even more discomfort or hassles. Continued interruptions necessary to urinate sometimes hampers late-night sleep, resulting in grogginess or irritability during daytime hours. Alcohol forces some people to experience low-quality sleep.

Compounding problems, excessive or even moderate caffeine consumption derived in everything from coffee and tea to soft drinks sometimes robs people of the ability of people to fall asleep at bedtime. People should avoid caffeine starting in the mid-afternoon or early evening.

Energy drinks packed with excessive amounts of caffeine fall within this category. Many such products also might excessively bolster alertness far longer than desired due to the amino acid taurine. When produced naturally within the body taurine helps regulate the blood's levels of salts and amino acids. Yet when taken in excessive quantities this substance can make falling asleep extremely difficult.

Avoid Three Foods before Bedtime

Following years of extensive research, scientists have identified three foods that people should be careful to avoid right before bedtime:

Chocolate: All forms of this, contained in everything from ice cream to candy bars and cups of cocoa, contain high amounts of caffeine and the stimulating amino acid tyrosine. Together, these substances make sleep almost impossible in many people.

Spicy foods, pizza and tomato sauce: These foods often cause various digestive disturbances including heartburn, symptoms that can hamper or stall sleep.

Preserved and smoked meats: These foods are loaded with the amino acid tyramine, which signals the brain's release of norepinephrine, which intensifies alertness. Food experts find high concentrations of tyramine in bacon, sausage, ham and smoked meats. Please avoid these as late-night snacks.

Late-afternoon exercise: Various studies have indicated to sleep experts that exercising in the morning is best for overall health. Detrimental results sometimes emerge from late-afternoon exercise, which tends to keep the metabolism in a high-overdrive mode, past the point of scheduled bedtime for most people.

To prevent such hassles, some doctors recommend completing any scheduled exercise at least three hours before scheduled bedtime. Doing that sometimes enables people to enjoy deeper and longer sleep.

For best results, consider varying your workout times and specific exercise routines in or to gradually pinpoint which overall routines work best for your particular metabolism. In fact, exercise routines in the mornings and early afternoon have consistently been shown to improve the quality of nighttime sleep.

Avoid nicotine: Many people know that nicotine derived primarily from tobacco products is a significant contributor to difficult-to-quit smoking habits.

From my professional experience, few people seem to realize that smoking often causes so much bodily stimulation that sleep becomes difficult. Various published reports also claim that nicotine can spark nightmares that interrupt sleep schedules.

Anyone who already smokes or chews tobacco should consider their potential or existing sleep problems as another reason to quit the habit, while the heightened danger of cancer should remain their primary motivator.

Teeth grinding: Called "bruxism" by medical experts, the frequent jaw clenching or grinding of the teeth is often blamed for sparking chronic sleep issues.

For such cases doctors need to identify and attempt to treat the underlying cause. Dull headaches and sore jaws upon awakening are among complaints of people suffering from bruxism.

Sadly, the general public fails to realize that this is a common sleep disorder. Dentists sometimes can determine if bruxism has caused a person's tooth damage.

The bodily damage intensifies among patients who also habitually chew their gums at night while grinding their teeth.

As a first line of potentially effective treatment after an initial bruxism diagnosis some doctors recommend such patients add chewing gum to their lifestyle habits. By doing so physicians hope the patient will relieve tensions that trigger tooth grinding.

A wide variety of other potentially effective treatments remain options, depending on each patient's specific needs or symptoms.

After medical professionals measure or build models of their jaws, some patients get specially built dental guards designed to prevent jaw grinding while asleep. Other potential treatments include relaxation strategies called "biofeedback," where patients learn to relax their muscles. Botox injections into the jaw are sometimes considered a last resort after other treatments fail.

Complete a Sleep Diary: One of the latest apparent fads might turn out as highly effective, creating daily sleep diaries in which the patient chronicles the previous night's sleep experience.

At a minimal cost that many patients might consider as "free," people suffering from sleep issues can keep a daily record of sleep issues or successes.

Among key topics to consider chronicling: "What activities were you involved during the evening prior to bedtime? What foods did you eat before bed? When was the meal and when was any exercise routine performed? Also, how well did you sleep? What interruptions were there, if any? And, how did you feel upon awakening in the morning."

If and when a doctor or sleep expert eventually reviews your diary, that person likely will want to know how many times you awakened if at all during the night. Great importance also is placed on how you feel during the day.

Your sleep expert or doctor might want to review your diary, looking for potential clues on a cause for your individual sleep issues.

Take action: Avoid tossing and turning in bed unnecessarily when and if you fail to fall asleep for an extended period at bedtime. When that happens, get out of bed and do something to pass the time.

Make use of a dream diary: You've probably heard of diaries that chronicle descriptions of dreams that are remembered on waking.

If you experience problems going to sleep, or difficulty sleeping as long as you want or need to, spend a few weeks keeping a sleep diary that records your sleep and sleep-related activities each evening.

Don't just lay there tormenting yourself: If you are tossing and turning for hours, unable to sleep, don't just lie in bed. This way you can strive to break any excessive anxieties or thoughts that might trigger insomnia.

Get up and do something useful. Read a book. Listen to music. Even watch television or surf the Internet.

Detox While Asleep

A Japanese product called BIO-MAT features rows of precious gems, Termalene and Amethyst. In nature, these emit far-infrared healing rays through your body to a depth of 6 inches to 8 inches. This energy mat has a number of benefits, including: improved circulation; relieves pain and joint stiffness; cleanses and detoxifies the body; accelerates injury recovery; improves metabolism; and stimulates immune functions.

6
Benefit From Sleep Relaxation Techniques

M any people suffering from sleep challenges such as insomnia, chronic snoring and sleep apnea first need to know that everything from mental tensions to anxiety and health problems might be causing the problem. A huge percentage of chronic sleep issues stems from a wide range of nervous system- or mind-related issues.

For people suffering from sleep problems, right away primary initial goals should be to address issues that are the likely cause of anxiety, depression or other issues that might rob the person's ability to rest.

Studies at various research laboratories and medical schools have chronicled what many health care professionals describe as the ideal self-help cognitive therapy strategies.

According to a 2007 article in *"Behavior Research Therapy,"* 19 people suffering from insomnia were treated with cognitive therapy for insomnia at the University of California, Berkeley, Sleep and Psychological Disorders Lab reported significant improvement. Researchers surveyed patients after three, six and 12 months of treatment. After a year researchers concluded that overall the patients experienced significant improvement in their ability to sleep at night and during the day.

Another study concluded that the results of using cognitive therapy were remarkable among 75 adults at an average age of 55 who had suffered insomnia symptoms at least 13 years, as reported by the "*Journal of the American Medical Association.*" As reported by the article, five researchers on the project concluded that such treatment "leads to clinically significant sleep improvements within six weeks and these improvements appear through six months of follow-up."

Among the most frequently used techniques for relieving stress, anxiety and mental tensions:

Autogenic training: People gradually learn to control their bodies' metabolisms, regulating everything from muscle tension and involuntary functions to blood pressure. A person successful at this usually can control the heart's rate.

Success hinges on controlling the "autonomic" component of the body's nervous system. Within healthy and even unhealthy individuals, the body has two distinct segments within the nervous system.

The parasympathetic nervous system regulates the body's digestion and the ability to efficiently rest, a key necessary component in the sleep process. The other component is vital to overall health, the sympathetic nervous system that regulates what doctors, scientists and psychologists call the body's natural "fight or flight" responses.

Researchers have been delving into the various critical aspects of these nervous systems including the impact on sleep since at least 1932. During the final decade leading up to World

War II a German scientist launched attempts to enable patients to efficiently balance and optimize functions of the sympathetic and parasympathetic nervous systems.

The overall process got labeled the "whole body" process, hinging on efforts to energize immunity and ignite healthy digestion while lowering blood pressure and calming the heart. To accomplish this, most experts recommend starting by quietly sitting in a meditative position while visualizing the entire body.

Begin by thinking of your arms as heavy and warm, before gradually thinking of the legs as having similar sensations. Each phase should be mentally repeated at least three times before proceeding to subsequent phases, such as my "legs are heavy and warm."

When the limbs start feeling as desired, begin thinking of your heartbeat as regular and calm. Experts in "autogenic training" claim that this strategy can work with some effort, largely because the mind ultimately controls the body.

Thus, for people experiencing sleep issues, the next phase after progressing through the limbs and the heart should focus on conveying positive messages about the body's digestive and sleeping processes. Some practitioners of this strategy report positive results when repeating these sessions over a period of time, usually weeks or months.

Biofeedback: In many ways this strategy is similar to autogenic training, although biofeedback usually involves simultaneously concentrating specific bodily areas that likely are causing to the individual's sleep issues.

A person with digestive issues that generate sleep problems

mentally focuses on commanding the body to fix or remove problems such as acid reflux symptoms.

Scientists or trained medical professionals connect the patient to electronic monitoring machines. These devices measure everything from heart rate and breathing to body temperatures. Through regularly scheduled practice, in a trial-and-error process, when successful the person can mentally command the body to relax or perform better.

During these sessions patients can easily see their various body measurements including the heart rate in "real time." Through steady and committed practice many patients successfully slow or energize their metabolisms as desired.

When under best-case scenarios involves sleep disorders, the patient concentrates on bodily areas that physicians have identified as the likely cause of such issues. A patient suffering from bruxism strives to relax the mouth and jaw. People who sleep too much on their backs strive to command the body to want to rest on other sides.

"This might sound like voodoo science, especially if you've never heard of such a process before," I tell some patients. "But many physicians and scientists insist that biofeedback has tremendous potential, backed by various research findings."

Besides directly targeting sleep issues, this strategy also can be used as an overall treatment effort to address symptoms caused by such problems. Among people with chronic sleep issues the various disorders or diseases that sometime cause resting problems include migraine headaches, fibromyalgia, neck pain, Parkinson's disease symptoms and hyperactivity disorder.

Behavior therapy: Sometimes called "cognitive behavioral therapy," this technique often targets people who suffer from a variety of issues including sleep problems, depression and anxiety.

Once again, I always stress that patients should only strive to work in conjunction with a physician or medical professional when attempting to address health issues. Nonetheless, once a patient learns fundamentals of behavior therapy, the patient can strive to use this strategy without assistance from anyone.

Experts insist that the key first step involves learning mental triggers that likely cause the mind to delve into dreary, dark dysfunctional patterns.

A common example involves taking a "catastrophic perspective," invariably visualizing worst-case scenarios for almost everything that happens in the person's life. Simultaneously, the person usually downplays or minimizes any good things that happen to them.

"How we think, and what we think about plays a huge factor in your quality of life," I tell patients. 'Thoughts can either destroy or strengthen your ability heal or to cope with extremely stressful situations."

Ultimately, the entire process of cognitive therapy hinges on this issue, primarily focusing on the potential "good" outcomes of situations rather than the "bad."

Mindful of this overall goal, from the start any person delving into cognitive therapy needs to create an action plan. Initial efforts involve generating "mental scripts" on what to think in certain situations, plus ways to eliminate "negative" behavior.

Guided Imagery: The power of the mind when striving

to manage sleep also becomes increasingly evident thanks to a process called "guided imagery."

"Essentially, we can make our daydreams come true," this strategy essentially implies. Once again, when employing this tactic, physicians, sleep experts and their patients strive to employ the great power of the mind in removing sleep issues.

To help put this into perspective, think of when you were a small child, teenager or young adult, perhaps prone to daydreaming. Such fantasies or goals at the time often became mentally powerful, perhaps enough to increase heart rates or form goose bumps.

Many of us know that merely thinking of a cozy tropical beach or the soothing sound of ocean waves somehow seem to generate such sensations and the resulting sense of pleasures within the mind. For some people, researchers say, the images and sensations of daydreaming become so powerful that the heart rate accelerates or the skin warms.

Such possibilities are so powerful that some researchers have delved into the positive potential such daydreaming or "guided imagery" can have on sleep issues.

Patients can appreciate the fact this is a low-cost potential treatment. Besides sleep issues, targets for treatment can include bodily diseases or conditions likely to trigger such problems.

Strategic daydreaming is so powerful that the effort can help reduce depression, stress or pain associated with side effects of cancer treatment, according to an American Cancer Society review of 46 studies on imagery and cancer. According to some published accounts, this tactic has occasionally been proven effective in reducing the size of cancer cells or killing tumors.

If true as many physicians and health care professionals believe, guided imagery can curtail a wide range of physical ailments or negative symptoms. This in turn, when effective, likely would increase the quality and duration of the patients sleep.

A 39-year-old woman was able to use guided imagery to turn a positive test for chicken pox virus into a negative result, and then back again; during the test period she envisioned the virus growing and then diminishing. These results were recorded by a research team at the University of Arkansas College of Medicine.

One of the best ways to learn the basics of such daydreaming or "guided imagery" is to scour the Internet or a vast range of books on the subject.

Hypnosis: Sleep experts believe that the body and particularly the mind reach a rather clear or hypnotic state during the stage immediately before sleep.

For more than 100 years, scientists, psychiatrists and standard-medicine doctors have labeled hypnosis a trance-like state. Oddly, a fact known only by a small handful of the general population, the brain often reaches a "blank" trance-like state even amid many standard awake-time, daytime activities.

The mystique and intrigue that hypnosis often generates is largely derived from this mental state's supposed "doorway into the soul." All along, various medical reports and scientific studies indicate that hypnosis and self-hypnosis can truly reduce or eliminate negative health symptoms—in some cases curing ailments.

Such positive possibilities can bring hope to many sufferers of sleep problems, at least according to various random, controlled and peer-reviewed sleep studies. Some reports claim that when effective, hypnosis can do everything from help heal bones and reduce anxiety to accelerating the body's natural healing process.

In one study, healing accelerated in specific areas of the bodies of burn victims, when they were told though hypnosis that such progress would occur in those regions. According to a report in the "*American Journal of Clinical Hypnosis*," among those patients burn healing was slower in other bodily areas.

Tai Chi: From the perspective of many Americans based on what they see on TV, people who engage in tai chi are usually Chinese seniors who participate in outdoor martial arts gatherings, methodically and slowly moving their limbs while standing.

Many westerners call this the "soft" martial arts, which strive to enhance longevity and overall health by training the body and mind relaxation techniques.

Scientists have been studying the potential benefits of such efforts, particularly whether tai chi improves the quality and duration of sleep.

According to various medical reports and research papers, the many potential benefits of tai chi can include increased bone density, accelerated rehabilitation of stroke victims and improvements in blood samples from people with Type-2 diabetes. Besides the possibility of improving cholesterol levels, reducing blood pressure and lowering risks from cardiovascular diseases, tai chi reportedly can generate natural antibodies and lessen tension headaches.

People can review a variety of Internet articles or books to easily learn how to incorporate tai chi into their lifestyles without joining group exercise regimens.

Qigong: Pronounced by English-speaking people as "chikung," this Chinese practice strives to maintain or achieve good health via proper visualization, breathing and posture. The treatment of insomnia is among health conditions health issues that qigong practitioners strive to control or eliminate.

Positive results from using qigong have been chronicled in dozens of medical studies. One of the best results involved a 58-year-old man, according to a 2004 report in the "Journal of Alternative and Complimentary Medicine."

In reporting for the publication, two professors listed a detailed report on the various physical improvements that the man experienced. Immediately before the research period commenced, the man suffered from a wide variety of ailments including allergies, asthma, elevated levels of prostate-specific antigens (PSA), and edema in the legs.

The research began as the man launched a several-month regimen of daily qigong therapy sessions. The publication reported that the man's blood pressure dropped to healthful levels, he lost 35 pounds and doctors were able to stop giving him medications.

A positive drop in this patient's pulse rate came as his asthma and allergies disappeared along with the edema and his PSA dropped to healthy levels.

A wide variety of Internet sites describe the basic and relatively easy process of how almost anyone can learn and start daily qigong regimens—particularly people who must address sleep issues.

Yoga: Perhaps one of the most effective methods of treating sleep issues and improving overall health involves this lifestyle practice.

Many people mistakenly believe that yoga is merely a form of exercise that involves a series of movements. Instead, this process strives to enhance overall health and vitality by uniting the body and mind.

People and societies in a variety of cultures have been practicing various forms of yoga since about 200 years before Christ. Some of yoga's first forms began in India, where lots of people began experimenting with various postures and breathing exercises.

As the centuries passed yoga practitioners began to claim that these efforts generated a positive impact on overall health.

Scientists in the 21st Century have conducted various studies in an effort to determine the validity of such claims.

In a six-week 2006 study of people suffering from coronary artery disease using yoga was found to improve lessen their symptoms, according to a report in the *"Clinical Cardiology"* journal. A 2004 study concluded that yoga relieved multiple sclerosis symptoms, according to the *"Neurology"* journal.

Perhaps just as impressive, as reported in *"Psycho-Oncology,"* researchers concluded that a wide range of physiological and physical benefits were enjoyed by breast cancer survivors who practiced yoga.

Most important from the perspective of people suffering from sleep issues, yoga also has been shown to address such problems while improving digestion and overall health.

7
The Magic of "Mindfulness"

Mental health experts including psychiatrists tell us that "mindfulness" entails the ability to always remain fully aware of our surroundings, usually without becoming unnecessarily disturbed by what occurs.

From the perspective of many experts, being fully mindful during a particular situation is tantamount to watching a train speed past you—while calmly and clearly observing each train car that passes, fully aware of each presence.

Just as important, while watching the train during an ideal mental state of complete mindfulness a person would always remain fully aware of any and all emotions, thoughts, sensations and opinions regarding the experience.

A person in an ideal mindful state refrains from placing blame, judging situations or rejecting others. Instead, the individual remains fully aware of everything that happens from moment-to-moment, fully cognizant of all thoughts or sensations. Although fully aware of each and every occurrence, the person refrains from being physically or emotionally disturbed by memories, perceptions, sensations, feelings and thoughts.

The opposite of "mindfulness," stress hails as a state where the individual allows worries about the present, past and future to dictate the mental state and bodily functions.

Dwelling on negative past events or the possibility of a dreary future often trigger the body's propensity to release natural hormones prone to undermining good health, such as cortisol and adrenaline.

When effective in managing sleep issues or other health problems, this technique often called "Mindfulness-based Stress Reduction" has been deemed potentially helpful in helping to treat or manage various diseases and negative health conditions.

Ultimately, putting yourself in a state of "mindfulness" can help the body eliminate underlying stress that either triggers or exacerbates various health issues.

This technique or treatment has sometimes been deemed powerful enough to eliminate such mental afflictions as obsessive-compulsive disorder, which causes a person to continually repeat activities in an effort to cope with extreme anxiety.

By eliminating various anxieties and mental tension, living in a state of mindfulness can go a long way toward improving the overall quality and duration of sleep.

Welcome Mindfulness Into Your Life

A professor emeritus at the University of Massachusetts, Jon Kabat-Zinn, PhD, played an instrumental role in introducing the possibilities of fighting disease and illness while reducing stress.

Researchers have identified two ways to bring mindfulness info your life, according to Kabat-Zinn, the Center for Mindfulness in Medicine, Health Care and Society's founding executive director:

Commitment: Set aside daily time to become still and silent by yourself in a quiet, meditative environment. While breathing deeply and slowly, concentrate on relaxing while mentally striving to put yourself into a state of well being.

Awareness: Continually strive daily to be and to remain fully aware of everything and everyone around you. This "informational mindfulness" technique stresses the importance of avoiding making any judgments, while refraining from becoming tense or anxious about any particular situation.

Kabat-Zinn believes this process and the results become easier and more effective after you have continued to engage in this process on a continuous basis.

"The most important thing to remember about mindfulness meditation is that it is about paying attention non-judgmentally in the present moment," Kabat-Zinn said. "We emphasize the present moment because that is the only time any of us are alive. The past is over, the future hasn't happened yet, and the only way we can effectively influence the future is by living fully and consciously in the moments in which we are actually alive, which is always NOW."

Benefit From Awareness Phases

The potentially positive impacts of mindfulness hinge on seven states of mind. Kabat-Zinn says these states combine to enable the body to regenerate:

Trust yourself: People sabotage the self-healing process when they fail to or refuse to trust their own feelings or bow to peer pressure.

Remain patient: Rather than rush to judgment or becoming anxious or depressed, allow yourself to observe unfolding events.

Non-Judgmental: Avoid becoming judgmental of others or of events, but instead remain an impartial witness.

Go With the Flow: Avoid striving to relax during potentially stressful situations, because doing so can actually trigger more stress. Instead, live moment-to-moment.

Blank Mind: Essentially react as if a child who has not yet formed opinions about how people "should" behave or the way events "should" transpire.

Let go: For most of us the mind tends to cling to how we've pre-programmed our feelings and thoughts to react negatively and positively to certain situations. Practitioners of mindfulness learn to refrain from making events, people or objects as less important or more important than they are.

Acceptance: Resting things that are and that you cannot change expends useless mental and physical energy, which also rob you of being fully present within the moment.

Hopefully, when and if these various states are used effectively, the various anxieties, stresses or physical ailments that spark sleep problems will significantly decrease or disappear.

Mindfulness Medication Techniques

Amid "mindless meditation" always assume the most comfortable position possible, such as lying on your back or sitting with the spine straight. Always relax all muscles within the body, particularly the shoulders—which you should let drop if sitting.

Then, close the eyes in order to avoid any unnecessary distractions.

"The easiest and most effective way to begin practicing mindfulness as a formal meditation practice is to simply focus your attention on your breathing and see what happens as you attempt to keep it there," says Dr. Kabat-Zinn.

Many people fail to realize until this process begins that the breathing process impacts or is effecting many different places throughout the body.

Some health professionals or people experienced with mindfulness medication suggest starting your concentrations on the nostrils. While focusing on this area of the body, feel each breath going through your nose. Then, observe your chest and belly expanding and contracting as you inhale and exhale.

Pay attention only to your breathing, and nothing else. Breathe naturally rather than forcing the inhale and exhale processes. By concentrating solely on your breathing, the mind will gradually leave any stressful thoughts. Do this at least 15 minutes daily for at least one week, steadily training the mind to avoid unnecessary concerns.

Remain cognizant of anything that distracts you for concentrating on your breathing. Later, mindfully concentrate on avoiding such distractions.

By this point you should start feeling comfortable, as if these meditations have evolved into a natural and comfortable part of your routine. With patience and practice as this daily routine continues for months you should start feeling comfortable concentrating on your breath without speaking, doing or saying anything.

Positive Study Results

A survey of articles detailing 38 medical research projects chronicled positive results when participants incorporated mindfulness into their sleep improvement efforts, according to the

University of Minnesota's Department of Family Medicine and Community Health.

According to the department's report as chronicled in a 2007 issue of *"Explore,"* "there is some evidence to suggest that increased practice of mindfulness techniques is associated with improved sleep and that mindfulness participants experienced a decrease in sleep-interfering cognitive processes."

8
Understand What Causes Insomnia

Just about any time someone suffers a sleep issue or fails to fall asleep, many people lacking medical training automatically label such conditions as "insomnia."

The very mention of the word seems as horrible as a ghost on Halloween, at least from the perspective of many people unfamiliar with this negative condition.

Sure enough, based on my experience and the observations of many other doctors, lots of people suffering from insomnia go into denial when learning they have the condition.

"Calm down and quietly attack the problem," I sometimes need to say. "First, accept that you have such a condition. Then, follow your doctor's advice in taking the best and the potentially most effective treatments in eliminating the condition."

Sadly, many insomnia suffers deny they suffer from that serious heath issue. Some patients also lack income necessary to get medical assistance.

By following my advice and general suggestions, many people can make significant progress on their own in identifying the likely causes of their individual sleep issues. Then, by following the general low-cost or "free" strategies that I recommend, insomnia sufferers sometimes can effectively address the issue without help from anyone but themselves.

Once again, at this point I feel the need to stress that no patient should ever attempt a thorough medial self-examination. Only a physician or highly trained medical professional can effectively make such a diagnosis.

Even so, when you've got a headache, for instance, a doctor never becomes necessary to proclaim that you're suffering from such a condition. Like many everyday people, when suffering from a headache you might take an aspirin or other low-dose, low-cost, pain-reducing analgesic.

Well, in many ways like an individual suffering from common aches and pains, you have a right to identify the likely cause of your apparent insomnia and then to take low-cost remedies or undergo inexpensive or "free" treatments.

Basic Evaluation Benefits

Huge amounts of literature and research reports on insomnia indicate that patients experiencing such symptoms should ask themselves these questions to determine the type of impairment they suffer:

Start time: Does the difficulty in sleeping commence at the beginning of bedtime when the patient wants to initially fall asleep? If so, this likely means the person fails to experience critical and necessary "delta sleep" or "slow wave sleep"—usually the deepest sleep of the night generally lacking rapid-eye movements or REM. The loss of slow wave sleep might be critical to a person's waking life, because the brain usually accumulates and catalogues the individual's short-term memory compiled from recent experiences. Increasing the dangers, according to numerous studies slow-wave sleep might decrease functioning of the body's sympathetic nervous system, while accelerating the parasympathetic nervous system. If true as some scientists believe, the loss of slow-wave sleep might have a negative snowballing effect on overall health. The malfunctioning of the sympathetic nervous system could hamper sleep efforts even more, while also hampering digestion—decreasing the body's efficiency in absorbing vital nutrients.

Re-awakening: Does the person suddenly and mysteriously re-awaken, perhaps a few hours after initially falling asleep for the night? Then, do attempts to fall back asleep become difficult or seemingly impossible? If so, the patient might regularly be losing the critical final phases of slow-wave sleep, while also losing some essential dream time. This could cause problems with the person's overall physical and mental health. Many researchers believe that the process of dreaming serves a vital role enabling the body and mind to cope with and address various stresses. An inability to dream could cause disorientation problems during periods of natural wakefulness.

Early risers: Perhaps just as critical, does the patient have a habit of awakening far too early in the morning after getting only four or five hours sleep? Does the patient have a tendency to rise out of bed for the day long before sunrise, especially after having stayed up late the previous night? If so, the individual likely would fail to receive the final dreaming stages that a healthy person without insomnia usually experiences. While more study might be necessary in this regard, such a loss might gradually emerge as detrimental to the person's overall long-term health. Whether such an early-riser habit might curtail or lessen a person's life expectancy has yet to be determined. Even so, from the view of many sleep experts such a loss in total average nightly sleep is likely a negative impact the overall health.

Sleep Diaries Become Increasingly Important

As briefly mentioned earlier, keeping a daily diary on your sleep issues and experiences can emerge as critical in helping doctors identify and address your specific health issues. When insomnia evolves into a serious problem rather than merely a minor sleep issue, the need for such a written chronicle intensifies.

A sleep diary will help you and your physician to easily list your overall sleep patterns. On a more intricate scale, with your sleep records the doctor should be able to pinpoint and target any negative habits or potentially destructive sleep-related instances.

Rather than merely chronicling what occurred during a span of just a few days, you should spend at least a few weeks chronicling your sleep patterns and habits. Doing so will give you and the physician a clearer view into your overall sleep-related health.

From the start of this diary process keep in mind that like a vast majority of people you might not initially be fully cognizant of your overall sleep patterns and habits. Some health professionals insist that an average person's overall propensity to sleep hinges on a mixture of everything from bodily sensations to emotions, thoughts and fantasies. Only after keeping a written record do likely sleep-issue triggers become apparent, such as:

Foods: Do nights of difficulty sleeping occur after eating certain foods or drinking specific beverages?

Emotions and moods: What are your moods and your overall thought process immediately before, during and after sleep? For instance, do you go to bed angry and awaken in a placid mood? Are you more irritable and less mentally sharp during daytime hours following nights when sleep was difficult or impossible?

Mental state: Keep a record of your mental state immediately before bedtime, followed by a description including any of that night's sleep issues. Also list your thought process before during and after sleep interruptions, including any worries pestering the mind.

Lifestyle choices: What did you do during sleep interruptions? Did you remain in bed trying to fall back asleep? List all the basics, such as tossing and turning, getting up to surf the Internet, or visiting the kitchen to grab a middle-of-the-night snack.

Potential distractions: Write about events or conditions that tended to awaken you or to prevent sleep, such a bright lights, uncomfortable temperatures or a noise such as nearby traffic, TVs, or loud neighbors.

Particularly if scheduling issues make compiling a daily diary difficult or seemingly impossible, use at least part of your late-night awake-time to jot down the events.

For many patients, the pathway to successfully identifying and addressing issues that they identified in the diary is to employ the numerous potential remedies described in previous chapters. The mind-calming, relaxation and mindfulness techniques can go a long way in positively addressing these specific issues.

9
Emotions Often Hamper Sleep

Thanks largely to intense study scientists have identified what researchers call the "Seven Deadly Emotions" most likely to generate insomnia.

This realization becomes critical when facing the fact that the chronic inability to sleep is actually a symptom of something else wrong, rather than the underlying problem.

Only a portion of overall insomnia cases stem from physical problems or ailments. So the blame usually should go to tensions, anxieties and emotions.

Thus, learning to ease mind and ridding the mind of pesky thoughts often can play a significant role in lessening or eliminating insomnia. Successful attempts at relaxation and calming the nerves can eliminate the need for potentially dangerous sedatives or sleep-inducing drugs.

With this understood you should thoroughly and carefully review the "Seven Deadly Emotions" to determine which if any are likely causes of your sleep problems which some experts call "insomnia emotions:"

Depression: This condition often involves a sensation of being trapped in a home or work environment, where the person might feel overly dependant on others amid a continually negative attitude or view about life.

Anger: Often accompanied by feelings of intense *frustration*, the patient might react as if having no control over situations that seem to overwhelm them. Such emotions send the mind into overdrive, keeping the brain and body in an agitated state.

Hopelessness: The individual feels as if there potential relief remains impossible, any way to escape destructive relationships or lifestyle conditions either at home or work.

Panic: Frustrations essentially reach the proverbial boiling point, as the person feels as if imprisoned in an environment or situation offering absolutely no opportunity for escape. The mind races with intense fear while any release seems impossible.

Anxiety: The person becomes overly anxious about one or more events in life, such as a job or a relationship. Concentrating too much on these issues can prohibit or interrupt sleep. Sometimes paying too much attention to the negative or scary events reported by the news media accelerates a person's emotions into overdrive, a point of "high anxiety."

Worry: Too much unnecessary time is spent pondering potentially negative outcomes or mentally striving to "solve" negative life events such as problems with the boss at work or conflicts with a spouse or loved one.

Meditate to Induce Sleep

Sleep expert John Selby has developed what he describes as a six-step medication technique specifically designed to relax the mind and body so that sleep can begin.

An overlying primary goal becomes the elimination or masking of the Seven Deadly Emotions, while also enabling the person to gradually feel fully relaxed.

Rather than merely scouring these stages listed below, people suffering from sleep issues including insomnia should fully review them several times.

Step 1: Get into the most comfortable position possible, preferably in bed. Shift your limbs until initially getting into the most relaxed bodily state. Then, focus the mind on breathing, particularly the air while slowly inhaling and exhaling. Continue concentrating on the air while allowing the eyes to close. This will help enable you to more fully concentrate on breathing, opening a pathway to avoid chaotic thoughts.

Step 2: While still concentrating on the air, steadily expand your sense of awareness regarding all the air going into and from your body. This way the mind can broaden its concentration to include the stomach and chest as those regions easily, naturally and effortlessly assist in drawing in and expelling air from the lungs. Gradually expand your concentration to include how the air flow creates movement throughout the body. Let this engulf and command your entire attention. This way, when and if other thoughts attempt to enter the mind, you can gently refocus the mind on breathing. Then focus, attention and practice you should experience an increased ability block outside thoughts.

Step 3: Continually relax while becoming aware of the jaw muscles, where tension sometimes becomes tense. Concentrate on relaxing this area along with the belly while exhaling. Always remain aware of the entire breathing process.

Step 4: Only after completing all previous steps, make the genital and pelvic region part of your expanded awareness as they meld with your breathing process. Briefly rotate forward and then resume a natural position, relaxing the belly muscles while exhaling.

Step 5: As your pelvis becomes increasingly relaxed, stop moving that area and then slightly move the toes—still fully mindful of all breathing. Briefly tense the toes before relaxing them. Then do the same with the fingers and hands, tensing before relaxing. Allow a feeling of relaxation to course through the entire body. As the day's tensions disappear, yawn, stretch and sigh after briefly tensing and relax the whole body while allowing every breath to send tranquility through your entire physical and mental being.

Step 6: Continually repeat mentally that "I'm ready to sleep," while remaining fully cognizant of relaxed natural breathing as air continually gets exhaled and inhaled.

Step 7: Start counting each breath if you have not yet started falling asleep. This often helps block or crowd away any thoughts that might try to arise. While exhaling think the word "sleep," while counting the latest breath as you inhale: "One, sleep...two, sleep..." Continue this until the mind welcomes sleep.

Be sure to memorize these basic, easy-to-remember steps before attempting them. Through time on a nightly basis this phased process can become part of your routine.

Remain dedicated to this free process which can emerge as powerful. For some people, this seven-step strategy becomes the only sleep-inducing strategy they need. Feel free to experiment and change or mix up these strategies as necessary to help address your own unique needs.

10
Additional
Sleep-Relaxation Tools

Various doctors, sleep experts and psychotherapists have
devised a variety of additional sleep-improvement methods.
Most strategies strive to release negative behaviors and thoughts,
decrease tension, anxiety and all of the Seven Deadly Emotions.

Among numerous sleep-reducing triggers and how to address
them:

Caffeine: Remain cognizant that caffeine, a natural stimulant
found in coffee, chocolate and some soda can remain in the body
for up to a day and a half. Some experts suggest that every person
who consumes more than 1.5 grams of caffeine daily should
consider gradually reducing their intake.

Darkness: Always strive to sleep in a dark area, because
otherwise your body might strive to naturally produce melatonin
that generates wakefulness. Unnecessary nighttime light also can
push the body's natural "sleep clock" off kilter.

Pro-active: Some people suffering from sleep problems
benefit by drinking beverages credited with inducing relaxation.
Chamomile and warm milk are often useful at bedtime in helping
to generate sleepiness.

Distractions: Do whatever you reasonably can to eliminate distractions, such as turning off the television beforehand or reading only away from bed. Scouring books, newspapers, magazines and notepads while in bed could keep you awake longer. Always maintain a quiet, relaxing bedroom environment.

The Two-Part Process

Numerous health experts tell patients that the sleep-relaxation process has two parts. First, work to release the body's muscular tension. Then, alleviate mental anxieties.

Various strategies are often mentioned, but for the most part these techniques involve variations of the seven-step process described in the previous chapter.

Any person who feels a need to delve further into successful bedtime relaxation techniques should remember that the words we choose to think can play a critical role.

In fact, specific thoughts and phrases that we chose to review or repeat quietly within the mind significantly impact our inner well-being. So whenever you must think, focus on calming and relaxing phrases rather than thoughts likely to increase anxiety or tension.

Both "negative" and "positive" phrases can send our bodies and minds in either of those directions. So, particularly during a stressful period in your life or following a particularly rough day, think of positive words and phrases.

Mentally repeating such words as "now," "quiet mind," "peace," "restful sleep" and "one" can emerge as powerful tools in gently commanding the mind to enter a tranquil state. Also, from the perspective of many people, quiet internal prayer can work wonders, such as thinking, "My God, please bring a quiet sense of peace to my mind, body and soul."

Get Creative

Rather than merely following what any particular book or video might tell you on the sleep-inducing subject, you should feel to "get creative" in developing helpful solutions.

Some people might choose to employ the seven-step sleep-inducing strategy during the middle of the day, or while they're in potentially stressful situations such as sitting in a doctor's office waiting room.

Using certain words or phrases during daytime hours can help generate a positive attitude likely to eliminate overall stress. These loving utterances in turn might help generate better nighttime sleep by reducing or eliminating tension.

As a key example, consider the case of Betty, a loving grandmother who recently lost her husband of 52 years to prostate cancer. Rather than cave in to loneliness and sorrow, Betty utters phases such as "great fruit" when scouring the grocery store produce section with her 8-year-old granddaughter.

"You've never liked ice cream, have you?" Betty teases the child, as they wander through the frozen-food section. Largely thanks to these tension-releasing behaviors, Betty sleeps relatively well at night.

Conversely, Betty's twin sister Bonnie, also recently widowed, tosses and turns alone in bed almost every night. Bonnie often scowls and uses negative, non-repeatable phrases even when in the presence of her grandchildren. Naturally, Bonnie's choice of gloomy phrases adversely impacts her body, her mind and her ability to sleep.

This comparison between Betty and Bonnie exemplifies the

awesome ability of our minds and bodies to go into the directions that we choose. Ultimately, for many people the overall quality of their sleep emerges as among the most significant results.

Destroy Your Sleeping Pill Habit

Addictions to powerful sleeping pills can be detrimental to the body and mind, while wreaking havoc on relationships, family life and the workplace.

Any person suffering from such debilitating addictions should acknowledge and admit to the problem while getting the assistance of a qualified health care professional.

A key strategy for kicking such habits, especially among those with mild addictions, involves engaging in tension-relieving and relaxing techniques such as those already described. For improved results, rather than merely focusing on the seven-step process, such patients can envision the many positive results of eliminating drugs from their lives.

Amid breathing and body relaxation in a meditative state, such patients can imagine never having to endure spending all their days and nights worrying about such pharmaceuticals.

Instead, amid meditation the person thinks of how much better life will be when free of chemical distortions. The mere thought of living free from pills enables some patients to better envision the pleasures of eating and benefiting from healthier foods.

By practicing and reviewing their meditative script beforehand, these patients often mentally envision their overall bodies becoming healthier as natural sleep patterns and times gradually return to their lives.

Physical and Lifestyle Improvements

While kicking sleeping pill addictions is undoubtedly difficult for many patients, researchers report that envisioning positive outcomes amid the meditative process can go a long way toward generating positive transitions.

For best results, many advisors recommend that patients envision a marked improvement in their overall lives. The mere notion of finally being able to naturally engage in bedtime without chemical dependence can help patients envision and eventually achieve such outcomes.

Positive Thinking Often Works

Traumatic life events such as car crashes, enduring wars, fear of starvation and witnessing sudden death can cause extreme anxiety that robs people of sleep.

Particularly in recent years, some of the most traumatic instances have received widespread public attention. After a through examination of a patient, doctors sometimes diagnose post-traumatic stress disorder or PTSD.

Fear, tension, anxiety and an extreme "survival mentality" often grips the lives of such patients. Sadly, many of these cases can last a lifetime while critically disrupting sleep unless professional intervention enables helps manage the condition.

Many PTSD patients in recent years have included U.S. military combat veterans from the wars in Iraq and Afghanistan. Media reports indicate the suicide rates among such people have been extremely high after they return home.

Even in cases where PTSD has not been diagnosed, horrific life events can cause serious damage to a person's psyche and thereby destroy or seriously disrupt or obliterate sleep patterns.

These severe anxieties can inflict people of any age. Young children whose parents die suddenly and tragically often suffer horrific nightmares that destroy the individual's ability to sleep. This becomes especially critical during a child's essential growth stage.

Overall these negative health conditions have imposed a formidable challenge to doctors and other health care professionals.

Thankfully, intensive and continual research has definitively shown that the age-old saying emerges as true that "the power of positive thinking actually works"—particularly among people desperately needing to effectively treat severe sleep issues.

Medical Evidence Backs These Claims

Steadily increasing numbers of separate research reports have identified what many practitioners of natural medicine hail as extremely beneficial. In essence, the results show that "positive imagery within the mind" often generates some of the best results.

Labeled "imagery rehearsal therapy" by many psychiatrists, psychologists and other medical professionals, this technique has been carefully studied in a variety of research efforts and reports. Among them:

Public need: "Imagery rehearsal therapy has received the most empirical support," which is significant because an estimated 8 percent of the population suffers from sleep disorders. These were the findings of two Sleep & Human Health Institute of New Mexico researchers, as reported in a 2006 issue of *"Behavior Sleep Medicine."*

Stress reduction: Among 168 women who had suffered severe nightmares generated by post-traumatic stress and sexual assault the positive results of creative imagery were significant, according to Sleep & Human Health Institute researchers. As reported in a "*Journal of the American Medical Association*" August 2001 issue, the researchers concluded that "imagery rehearsal therapy is a well-tolerated treatment that appears to decrease chronic nightmares, improve sleep quality, and decrease post-traumatic stress disorder symptom severity."

Similar results: At Oxford University in the United Kingdom, creative imagery used in a study of 41 insomnia patients showed that the efforts helped distract the mind from negative issues. In one of three sets of groups that these people were divided into, creative imagery enabled participants to fall asleep faster. As reported in the British journal "*Behavior Research and Therapy*" in March 2002, "the success of the imagery distraction task is attributed to it occupying sufficient 'cognitive space' to keep the individual from re-engaging with thoughts, worries, and concerns during the pre-sleep period."

Results such as these come as good news to sufferers of light or severe insomnia sufferers who have been unable to afford professional treatment. Positive-imagery techniques also can benefit people who had been unaware that their insomnia has likely imposed extreme danger to their overall health.

Even people who have suffered from mild sleep disorders could benefit, particularly if they consistently strive to engage in positive imagery. A wide variety of online articles and books on this specific technique are available online.

11
Whether Sleeping Pills are "Good" or "Bad"

Even among people who strive to avoid hearing this, the truth is that Mother Nature does not consider pill popping as natural or effective for everything that ails us.

You should be weary of any person, doctor or pharmaceutical company that says otherwise, especially if the medication involves sleep issues.

To their own detriment in many cases, many people consider ingesting pills and particularly sleep medications as natural—especially in instances where they have already made this a habit.

Rather than wanting us to rely on pills, within healthy humans Mother Nature has biological systems that make sleep regular, natural and necessary.

Even so, many people feel they need to resort to sleeping pills, particularly individuals who have failed to correct the problem with other methods.

If you now take sleeping pills on a regular basis, you can decide whether to stop the habit by first asking yourself several basic questions:

Behavior: After deep thought and inner reflection while refusing to go into denial, do you consider such behavior as abnormal?

Habit: Do you often or at least regularly take sleeping pills out of habit, even in instances where you do not particularly have any problem falling asleep?

Risks: Do you know of any risks imposed by the pills that you take, and do those dangers outweigh the potential benefit?

Addictive: Is the particular medication addictive in nature or habit forming? Or, perhaps, could you be addicted to the mere habit of taking the pills?

Ultimately, in determining whether to try to stop such a routine a patient needs to decide whether the drugs are causing more harm than good. Other factors to consider include potential emotional conflicts.

Pills, Dangers and Emotions

If this controversy were a hit TV show, it might be called "Sleepers Gone Wild."

Besides the participants, most of them insomnia sufferers, the key conflicts featured prominently on every episode would hinge on pills, the potential dangers and emotions.

Through the past century many celebrities have suffered the ultimate consequence of death when engaging in this extremely risky reality show.

Sleeping pills or sleep medications have been blamed as primary factors in the deaths of Elvis Presley, Marilyn Monroe, Michael Jackson and numerous other celebrities.

Sadly, huge numbers of everyday "regular" people who never make headlines have suffered similar fates.

Many people might want to blame doctors for prescribing such powerful medications. Some individuals highly addicted to particular sleeping pills obtain those drugs illegally on the black market.

An unknown percentage of deadly instances involve physicians who over-prescribe such medications.

At least from my perspective as a seasoned medical professional, some doctors strive to use a warped form of logic in attempting to rationalize why they prescribe such pills. Lots of these physicians wrongly consider "real nature" as part of an insomnia patient's problem.

Instead, those doctors should be trying to identify the underlying cause of each person's sleep issue, and then strive to generate effective remedies to address triggering factors that rob the person of an ability to sleep.

Blame Emotional Issues

Besides pain from injuries or from diseases like cancer, much of the time sleep problems that doctors strive to address with drugs actually stem from emotional issues.

Doctors who merely strive to address the sleep-loss symptom by prescribing sleep-inducing pills are providing a disservice to their patients and to society as well.

A vast array of potentially dangerous or addictive sleep drugs are produced by major pharmaceutical companies that generate enormous profits from such sales.

The list of these extremely dangerous medications is seemingly endless. Some of most dangerous brand-name or generic-named sleep drugs include: Amytal, Nembutal, Phenobarbital, Seconal, Dalmane, Luminal, and Tranxene.

Even among otherwise healthy patients, particularly those

addicted to the medications, accidental fatal overdoses emerge as an extreme danger. The potentially worst and most dangerous of these pills can only be legally obtained via prescription.

I refer to the most dangerous sleep medications as an overall group as "knockout drugs," which should only be issued to patients only as a last resort.

Powerful Drugs Ruin Sleep

Rather than improve or eliminate sleep issues, the long-term use of high-power sleep medicines generally reduces or damages the ability to benefit from such natural activity.

Such medications usually pass or override the body's natural sleep cycles. The patient experiences a radically different resting experience than nature provides.

Whenever they're honest with themselves or with others, people who regularly ingest such pharmaceuticals usually complain of feeling as if drugged when they awaken. Common complaints range from "I'm feeling comatose," to "I'm still sleepy."

Invariably, the person feels far from well-rested. To the contrary, throughout the day these patients invariably feel sluggish, extremely tired and irritable or moody.

Needless to say, the patient's overall situation becomes far from healthy. This pattern remains until the person dies, becomes critically ill and therefore unable to take the drugs, loses access to the pharmaceuticals or manages to quit the habit.

Until this pattern ends, the person usually fails to receive adequate amounts of healthy dreams, many or most masked or blocked by the drugs.

With these various dangers and potential pitfalls in mind, anyone who considers starting such medications should remain extremely skeptical. Remember that drugs usually treat symptoms rather than the causes. The challenge multiples when unnatural treatments and especially powerful drugs can trigger additional health issues.

Understand Sleep Drug Categories

Particularly among people who lack medical knowledge or education, the maze of available sleep drugs can seem challenging or even confusing.

Perhaps more eager to generate profit than to actually help people, huge pharmaceutical companies nicknamed "Big Pharma" have developed numerous categories of such medications.

The varieties and brands of specific pills is so voluminous that even some highly experienced doctors need to refer to their "drug bible"—formally called the Physicians Desk Reference or PDR. This voluminous publication updated annually lists all primary drugs that have been authorized for licensed physicians to prescribe.

Greedy Big Pharma charges up to $5 for a single pill, or even much more. Eager for relief of their problem, some desperate patients are willing to pay for over-priced drugs that might tend to do them more harm than good.

Sadly, based on my professional observations during more than 40 years as a practicing physician, I can testify that many insomnia patients are never told that they might benefit from potentially effective treatments that avoid drugs.

The many dozens of high-power medications generate

different impacts. So, patients using such pharmaceuticals need to clearly understand the basics of each category:

Benzodiazepine: Sometimes hailed as "psychoactive" or even "psychedelic," these drugs can generate hallucinations and even an almost unshakable dependence. Such drugs primarily target the body's critical central nervous system, partly in an effort to reduce anxieties that sometimes hamper or prevent sleep. Potentially severe and life-changing negative side effects can emerge, including the development of long-term amnesia, irritability, nausea and even depression. A vast range of drugs within this category includes Ativan, Xanax, and Valium.

Non-Benzodiazepines: Particularly among patients using these drugs for extended periods, psychological and physical side effects are among potential dangers. Some long-term users reportedly suffer from a degradation of cognitive abilities, amnesia and reduced memory functions. The most prevalent brand names within this sector include Lunesta, Sonata, Zolnod and Ambien.

Anti-Depressants: Amazingly, some doctors choose to prescribe anti-depressants. Rather than strive to identify and address a patient's underlying cause of sleep disorders, these physicians employ anti-depressants which have tranquilizing, sedative effects. By generating sleep-like conditions among patients, the health care professional avoids the person's underlying health issue. Prescribing such drugs for the treatment of sleep disorders or problems is done so "off-label." The pharmaceutical companies produce these drugs such as Desyrl, Elavil, and Risperdal for health issues other than sleep.

The Booming Sleep-Drug Market

Within today's increasingly stressful and hectic society the number and types of sleep drugs produced by Big Pharma has been rapidly growing.

Among these is the Rozerem sedative that some sleep experts consider safer because this drug releases natural melatonin produced naturally in healthy people. Remember, melatonin naturally plays a critical role in regulating the body's internal clock or "circadian rhythm."

Medical experts formally list Rozerem marketed by Takeda Pharmaceuticals North America as the first in a new class of sleep-agent drugs. According to various published reports and studies, the potential or existing benefits of Rozerem, especially when compared to other sleep medicines, include:

Addiction: This has not been shown to cause physical or psychological dependence.

Targets: Attacks insomnia, particularly among patients who complain of difficulty falling asleep.

Function: Integrates well with the biological receptors within the body and brain critical in the regulation of sleep and resting patterns.

In October 2008, the U.S. Food and Drug Administration, commonly called the FDA, approved Rozerem for insomnia treatment and especially for patients with problems falling asleep.

Critical Summary

Ultimately, doctors and sleep experts need to understand and to tell patients that all drugs fail miserably in treating insomnia. Any physician who has carefully followed the issue knows that clinical research has proven indisputably that pharmaceutical products other than those made from natural substances do nothing to "fix" the underlying cause. Although drugs might seem to induce temporary relief, the underlying causes of sleep disorders must be treated in order to generate potential long-term relief.

12

Determine the Amount of Sleep You Need

Right away you need to forget society's widespread notion that every person needs exactly eight hours of sound sleep nightly in order to achieve and maintain good health.

To the contrary, each person has his or her own unique sleep needs. The reasons for these differences range from variations in metabolism, hormones and overall health.

Hereditary factors also might play a significant role. This is coupled with a person's age. Sleep patterns, times and quality vary depending on each person's particular stage in life at any given time.

At least one thing is clear regarding sleep among all ages, body types and metabolisms. Scientists know that people do not necessarily experience the good and healthful sleep that they need, just because their eyes remain closed for extended periods.

Good overall health hinges on how much of the person's sleep time involves extremely deep and rejuvenating "delta sleep."

During this stage the brain generates delta waves, while the body and mind transition into the rapid-eye or REM sleep mode. Both of these essential sleep phases are critical to generating and maintaining overall good health, enabling the immune system and the endocrine system and critical organs to work naturally and effortlessly at maximum capacity.

People often complain of feeling groggy or disoriented when suddenly awakened from delta-stage sleep. This should signal to any person suffering from sleep issues that their goals should include getting as s much high-quality delta sleep as possible. Meantime, the REM sleep phases, which generate an active dream state throughout the night, are essential to the patient as well.

Interesting Needs

Primary, basic and natural amounts of both REM sleep and especially delta sleep are critical for people to function well mentally and physically during the daytime.

Some scientists believe that any individual, who seems to need relatively little sleep at night, perhaps seven hours or less, probably skips the natural step-by-step sleep phases.

Through the night, starting from bedtime most people gradually evolve into increasingly deeper phases of sleep. Anyone who sleeps for only short periods at night zips almost immediately past the delta stage into REM sleep.

Overall, health care professionals seem increasingly intrigued that a small percentage of people seem to need much less sleep than the bulk of the population.

Some researchers have suggested that perhaps people needing little sleep nightly somehow have an innate, inbred ability to thrive mentally and physically with significantly less delta-stage sleep than most people.

Unique Conditions Abound

For now scientists seem to lack conclusive evidence on why this extremely small percentage of the population apparently lacks any need for extensive delta-wave sleep.

Perhaps heredity plays a significant factor. Or, maybe these individuals somehow evolved differently than most of us for unknown reasons.

Various reports and historic accounts claim that the iconic inventor Thomas Edison remained vibrant and creative while needing only five hours night sleep. By contrast, at least if various reports are to be believed, the genius Albert Einstein who developed the Theory of Relativity needed at least ten hours nightly sleep to remain mentally vibrant.

Although a small segment of the overall population thrives mentally and physically with little sleep, the vast majority of us are settled with greater needs in that regard. Among some sleep requirement categories that health experts generally agree upon:

Infants: From 16 hours to 18 hours sleep daily on average.

Teens: Around nine hours daily, longer than most adults because at this stage people undergo growth spurts that require vital natural growth hormones produced during rest.

Pregnancy: Especially during the first three months, expecting women usually need several hours more of daily sleep than they would otherwise get on average.

Average Daily Sleep Times

Although some minor disputes remain on the issue, scientists and researchers generally fail to list a specific average sleep-time requirement for the adult population.

Everything here rests on the fact that each individual has unique needs in this regard.

With this clearly understood, the question arises, "What about you? How much sleep do your body and mind require on average on a daily basis?"

On your own without help from a medical professional the answers might appear after asking yourself some basic questions. Among them:

Mornings: What is your mental condition upon awakening most mornings? Do you feel wide awake, and mentally vibrant? Or, do physical and mental sluggishness dominate?

Daytime: Do you suddenly or unexpectedly feel drowsy during the middle of the day, particularly during the afternoons? Does your mental vigor sag, after seeming fairly normal or even sharp during the mornings?

Atmosphere: Do your job or your personal relationships suffer following nights where you do not seem to sleep long enough. Yet do your work and relationships somehow improve on days when you go to bed earlier than usual or sleep late?

Bedtime: Do you become increasingly grouchy during the evenings or right before regular bedtime, even after getting adequate amounts of exercise and healthy meals throughout the day?

A "yes" answer to one or more of these questions might emerge as a likely signal that perhaps you lack sufficient nighttime sleep on an average day.

Insufficient Sleep Shortens the Lifespan

The cold, hard, indisputable facts backed up by a variety

of intense medical studies indicate as suggested earlier that insufficient sleep usually shortens a person's lifespan.

The overall dangers throughout society become increasingly clear. Surveys show that insufficient sleep impacts nearly one third employed people within the United States. That's up from about a quarter of the population 10 years earlier.

Perhaps today's fast-paced work environments that seem to place increasingly intense demand on workers and executives triggers tensions that hamper sleep patterns.

Indeed, at least one out of very four people surveyed confessed to driving while sleepy, particularly in instances where they already have difficulty sleeping. If true, the lack of sleep might hamper good judgment, leading to poor and dangerous decisions.

Motorists need to remain fully cognizant at all times of the disturbing fact that a significant percentage of people driving at any given time while overly drowsy, particularly at night. Sane, sober and well-rested drivers need to remain on the lookout for sleep-deprived motorists.

You also should pull off the road and rest even while sober if your vehicle drifts into other lanes, your eyelids feel heavy, you start yawning, or you have problems holding your head up.

Ineffective or extremely dangerous strategies of correcting such problems range from drinking caffeine that takes up to 30 minutes to enter the bloodstream to keeping the vehicles windows open.

Instead, rather than striving to continue driving while drowsy, you should pull to the side of the road into a safe place and sleep at least 15 minutes to 20 minutes.

To do otherwise would be to risk becoming a "grim statistic." Authorities estimate that 1,550 people die yearly in vehicle accidents due to sleep issues. The data indicates that sleep-related crashes injure at least 71,000 people yearly.

Excessive Sleep Imposes Dangers

Depression is often listed as among the most apparent causes of people sleeping too much or far more than necessary.

One of the most compelling studies indicated a connection between mortality rates and sleep duration, as reported in the "Journal of the American Geriatric Society."

The publication's October 2010 issue chronicled a study of 3,820 people older than age 59. Researchers strived to determine any link between sleep duration and early death.

Following an eight-year stretch beginning in 2001, the researchers compared people who sleep seven hours nightly to those who slept eight hours to 11 hours or even longer.

The results indicated that people who slept less lived longer. Similar results emerged among people who reported themselves in good health as they joined the study.

All along, the focus of most sleep experts targets issues involving people who sleep too little. Yet conclusions such as those in the geriatric study should motivate people who sleep nine or more hours nightly to get a thorough medical exam as soon as possible.

Serious Illness Impacts Sleep

Just about everyone has experienced a serious illness such as the flu at least sometime in life. Through personal experience, almost all of us know that critical health issues often hamper or block the ability to sleep—or put such activity into overdrive.

Such instances serve as vivid examples of the vital interplay between our overall health and sleep. Many people suffering early stages of the flu start feeling drowsy, as the brain orders the body's vital immune system to click into overdrive.

Much of the time when such health emergencies erupt the ability, duration and quality of sleep become an essential and effective bodily weapon clearing a pathway toward eventual recovery.

Particularly during sleep, our bodies are better able to develop necessary invader-fighting antibodies.

Extensive rest also enables the pituitary gland within the brain to kick into overdrive, generating essential growth hormones to help the body gain or retain strength. Sure enough, for most viruses or injuries plenty of bed rest and particularly sleep become essential, often while striving to drink an appropriate and ample amount of clear fluids.

This is largely why for many generations doctors, including in classic movies produced through the 20th Century, have been known to tell patients: "Get plenty of bed rest, and be sure to drink lots of fluids."

Essential Natural Hormones Help

Doctors have known for many generations that essential natural hormones or other substances created within the body while fighting disease often help to generate sleep.

One of the most essential key players here are cytokines, powerful natural immune-boosting chemicals within the body that make the person sleepy.

This is Mother Nature's creative and essential way of helping the body conserve energy. When the entire process works naturally and in scheduled phases, the immune system musters up enough necessary vigor to whip viruses or to accelerate the creation of vital bodily chemicals and white blood cells necessary to help repair wounds.

The opposite sometimes occurs when we lack sufficient sleep. When that happens chances increase that the immune system will fall off balance, stall or even fail.

The destruction or degradation of the immune system can and often does often lead to the development of serious diseases and eventually death. With this clearly understood by you, the need to get healthful sleep should become increasingly apparent.

Heed These Compelling Study Results

Disjointed and unhealthy sleep patterns shorten your lifespan by igniting disease, according to an increasing number of scientific studies. Among a handful of the many shocking or mind-opening examples:

Death: A 2009 report in the "Journal of Sleep Research" chronicled numerous studies indicating that people who sleep at least nine hours nightly have an increased risk of death, as compared to people who slept from seven hours to eight hours nightly.

Danger: Along with the development of bodily evidence of cardiovascular disease, blood pressures increased and heart rates accelerated among people in a test group whose sleep was restricted to less than four hours nightly, according to a 1997 report issued in "Hypertension."

Diabetes: The danger of diabetes erupted among patients restricted to less than four hours of nightly sleep, by slowing the body's ability to tolerate glucose, according to a medical study reported in 1999 by "Lancet."

Inflammation: Sleeping less than four hours nightly also was shown to increase inflammation within the body. The sleep depravation impacted the body's C-reactive protein, a bodily marker known to increase the risk of coronary artery disease, according to a 2004 report in the "*Journal of the American College of Cardiology.*"

Obesity: A separate study reported in a 2004 by the "*Annals of Internal Medicine*" indicated that sleeping less than four hours nightly can accelerate the appetite. This condition can trigger the onset of weight gain leading to obesity.

Hypertension: Blood pressure is likely to increase in people deprived of sufficient rapid-eye movement sleep, potentially leading to critical health issues, according to a report in the February 2010 issue of the "*Journal of the American Medical Association.*"

Alzheimer's disease: Sleep disorders potentially represent a dementia symptom, triggering the progression of mild cognitive impairment that leads to such disease, according to a March 2010 report in the "Journal of Nutrition Health."

Immunity: A study reported in a 2002 issue of the "*Journal of the American Medical Association*" indicated that young adults had less than half of the antibody response of healthy people—when injected with flu vaccine immediately after four nights of abnormal sleep.

13
Benefit from Natural Sleep Aids

Natural remedies should always become your highest priority when striving to treat sleep issues.

This strategy makes the most sense. Healthy people always sleep naturally, especially when health issues or outside factors fail to trigger events that awaken them.

Sadly, the huge pharmaceutical industry spends perhaps billions of dollars in yearly advertising to make the overall public believe otherwise.

Consumers who insist on natural remedies have to ignore the dangerous advice given by Big Pharma advertisements and by mainstream doctors. For many patients doing so can emerge as challenging. After all, why not listen to the so-called experts.

The potential danger intensifies for average consumers. The vast majority of people seem to lack any inkling that natural remedies are far more preferable.

Determined to help bring the public vital information regarding the benefits of natural remedies, many of the best natural sleep aids can be considered.

Like similar professional practitioners of natural remedies, as a licensed homeopath when a patient's examination results warrant such action, I prescribe or recommend small amounts of substances found in nature.

Within a variety of cultures through many generations people embracing natural medicine have tested and proven the positive impacts from such treatments. Mother Nature provides effective and harmless plant-based substances proven effective in addressing everything from pain to sleep issues.

As a key example, did you know that aspirin is derived naturally from the bark of willow trees? This is just one of many hundreds of natural substances that homeopaths have helped identify as highly effective treatments for a variety of health problems.

Important List of Natural Options

The following list of essential natural treatment options should be considered for sleep issues, especially after other non-drug tension relieving tactics have failed.

Many of these products and herbs, usually available primarily via homeopaths, also prove effective when used in conjunction with natural strategies such as "mindfulness" and meditation.

A comprehensive list of these substances could fill volumes. Here are just some of the basics that I often consider as initial options, depending on each patient's needs:

Silica: Often praised for its ability to enhance sleep, it's derived from flint.

Cocculus: Derived from 11 species of woody vines and shrubs, often from tropical climates this substance hailed as "moonseed" helps people who complain: "I'm too tired to sleep."

Sulphur: Among the basic chemical elements that many of us learned about in high school, this natural element has been praised for insomnia sufferers—especially among people who fail to get sufficient exercise.

Herbs: Most effective when found or grown naturally, the many varieties deemed effective in helping sleep include Saint John's wort, chamomile, valerian and passion flower.

Lycopodium: Derived primarily from creeping cedar and ground pines, this is among plant-based substances often deemed highly effective at inducing sleep.

Arsenicum album: This is often prepared by diluting arsenic trioxide, usually to the point where the solution contains only a few or even no remaining molecules. Sometimes prescribed for treating arsenic poisoning, arsenicum album can also help sleep issues.

Nux vomica: Also known as the "strychnine tree," "poison nut," or various other names, the natural products from this deciduous tree found primarily in Southeast Asia. Besides the treatment of hangovers, it's also deemed effective for insomnia.

Ignatia amara: Native to the Philippines and sections of China, this pear-shaped fruit can work wonders for insomnia sufferers. Although sometimes used as rat poison due to its limited amounts of strychnine, when used in extremely minute quantities this substance is effective in treating a variety of conditions including depression and grief.

Appreciate Human Growth Hormones

The cast of critical biological players gets formidable assistance from another key natural internal substance mentioned earlier, "human growth hormones" or HGH.

Described in greater detail in several of my other hot-selling books, HGH gets formed within the body largely as a result on melatonin's impact on the "body clock."

Within healthy people, particularly individuals benefiting from healthful sleep, melatonin triggers the natural production of HGH by the pituitary gland.

As people age, their bodies tend to generate higher levels of serotonin than melatonin. This imbalance sometimes generates health issues including sleep disruptions, particularly within mature people. Besides sexual dysfunction, potential symptoms range from sleep apnea to the possible development of Type II diabetes mellitus.

Needless to say, the dominance of serotonin within the bodies of older people often emerges as a precursor for significant, life-threatening or potentially deadly health issues.

The proverbial "hidden bullet" here stems from the loss or serious decrease in melatonin, which when generated at optimal levels within healthy people serves a giant role in the body's overall healing and immunity processes.

14
Appreciate Melatonin

The naturally produced substance within the body mentioned earlier, melatonin, boasts anti-aging benefits thanks largely to its ability to regulate the "body clock" or circadian rhythm.

Homeopaths and many consumers consider inexpensive melatonin pills as far more beneficial and effective than high-priced and extremely dangerous Big Pharma drugs.

Melatonin plays a critical and essential role in enabling the body to generate critical delta-stage sleep needed for optimized physical and mental health.

More specifically, many people benefiting from melatonin pills appreciate the fact this works wonders in helping to regulate and assure the body's 24-hour performance.

Besides sleep, the many secondary and important functions that melatonin directly or indirectly plays a role in include digestion and alertness. A clear and sharp mind is the pathway to survival and to increasing the probability of thriving economically, socially, health-wise and within interpersonal relationships.

In the human body, melatonin is derived from the pineal gland, a sub-centimeter organ within the center of the brain. Engulfed in a rich supply of blood, the pineal gland generates massive quantities of serotonin, which essentially serves as a thermostat regulating body functions.

Generated by serotonin, melatonin plays a critical role in managing the body's energy. Its vital functions include regulating the testosterone sex hormone and regulating stress levels.

Anyone aware of these essential functions that melatonin provides can appreciate the importance of sleep in our lives, plus the function this substance plays in the anti-aging and good-health processes.

Understand Melatonin's Many Benefits

Besides managing the body's "biological clock," generating healthful sleep, boosting immunity and timing good digestion, melatonin also helps to battle or block dangerous and potentially carcinogenic "free radicals."

A free radical is an unpaired atom within molecules or substances that are not already paired up with or linked to other atoms. When left unchecked, free radicals can lead to severe health conditions or life-threatening diseases such as cancer.

Along with various hormones and biological structures including natural killer-class blood cells, melatonin directly or indirectly battles free radicals within the brain and spinal fluid.

These continual wars that we're mentally unaware of often erupt when free radicals attempt to invade the body by attaching to water, food or various toxic substances that we come into contact with.

Unless and until melatonin and the body's other protective mechanisms successfully block or destroy free radicals, these invaders can adversely accelerate the aging process.

Our appreciation for melatonin should increase multi-fold upon realizing that our brains likely would suffer a decrease in cognitive ability without the extraordinary role melatonin plays in defending that organ from free radicals.

In at least one laboratory study conducted in at the University of Texas Health Center in San Antonio, melatonin enabled rats to ward off cancer. First, researchers subjected the rodents to carcinogens.

Then, a portion of rats within the overall test group were given melatonin. Impressive results emerged when researchers found that the rats receiving melatonin suffered 50 percent less genetic damage than rodents not given the substance.

Many People Benefit

Besides those regularly suffering from sleep issues while remaining at home, the many people benefiting from melatonin pills include frequent travelers such as commercial airline personnel and night-shift workers.

The formidable benefits of melatonin are universally deemed so powerful that many airline companies recommend that their employees take melatonin to alleviate or to minimize the potentially adverse symptoms of jet lag.

Globe-trotting people who frequently travel to vastly different time zones often refrain from experiencing excessive grogginess or a sense of mental instability when they ingest melatonin.

Indeed, particularly when taken in optimal situations melatonin can sometimes effectively aid in resuming or maintaining healthful, natural sleep levels.

Particularly for those who desire the anti-aging attributes of good sleep, melatonin pills could serve as a key factor in triggering desired results. Mice in a Russian study that received melatonin lived 25 percent longer than similar rodents not given the substance.

Melatonin Secrets

Melatonin is so powerful that anyone using the pills and particularly seniors should avoid ingesting them at least one day per week. This becomes necessary in order to allow the pineal gland to continue the uninhibited production of the substance.

Among other strategies or methods that I recommend when taking melatonin:

Seniors: Start by taking lower doses of just 1-3 milligrams at bedtime if you're over age 49. Those who choose to take melatonin should do so about every other day, but no more than six days per week.

Seasons: Those taking melatonin pills should realize that when made naturally within the body the levels of this substance often click en tandem with seasons of the year. This occurs when daylight extends in summers and contracts during winter months. Adjust the amounts of pills taken, depending on how sleep you feel or that you need to become during any particular season.

Pregnancy: Pregnant women should avoid taking melatonin, to avoid any unnecessary disturbances or hormonal changes inside the unborn child within the embryo and fetus stages.

Doses: Generally, adults of within normal size ranges and of fairly good health can easily tolerate 10-20 milligram melatonin doses. Some people prefer taking these pills at bedtime.

Sleep apnea: Big Pharma has been unable to produce any high-priced drugs that I consider effective in directly treating sleep apnea. Some studies suggest that people suffering from sleep apnea may benefit from doses of 10-20 milligrams of melatonin at bedtime.

Ingredients: At least one fairly new product, Somnapure, contains sleep ingredients that include melatonin, plus various herbs including passionflower and chamomile.

Cancer: Integrative oncologists have used higher doses of melatonin in the 20-30 milligram range successfully in prostate, breast and other cancers as adjuvant hormonal therapies.

15
Sexual Benefits

B esides being healthy, fun and potentially energizing when engaged in between consenting adults, sex can generate powerful, healthful and anti-aging sleep.

During and after sex and particularly in the wake of spectacular orgasms the bodies of both genders often benefit from a sharp drop in blood pressure. This reaction is usually far more prominent in men, who have a well-deserved reputation for sleeping after sex.

When given a choice of whether to take dangerous drugs or to engage in consensual adult sex in order to induce sleep, the wise decision mirrors what the famed Broadway song from "Annie Get Your Gun" says, "Doing what comes naturally."

Even people skittish at the mention of sex might benefit significantly from learning just some of the basic sleep-related results that orgasms can generate. Among them:

Depression: Sex can clear the mind at least temporarily scrubbing away troublesome thoughts that cause depression, a known sleep inhibitor.

Stress: When done naturally, beautifully and sometimes widely erotic in nature, sex can wipe away bodily and mental stress that might otherwise hamper sleep.

Mood: Various hormones including endorphins released energetically into the body during and immediately after sex can sharply elevate the mood, obliterating or maxing one of the biggest killers of sleep—anxiety.

Impotence: Any lack of desire for sex or a form of sexual disorder, conditions that often impact older men, can sometimes hamper passion that would lead to physical intimacy. Anyone experiencing such symptoms—yet still eager to benefit from the anti-aging and sleep-inducing benefits of sex—should seek the care and guidance of medical professional or sex therapist.

Pain: Sleep can induce an analgesic effect throughout the body, sometimes lessening physical pains that might otherwise hamper recovery.

Insatiable: Having more frequent sex should become a goal of many consenting adults and particularly seniors, especially upon learning that various studies show that older people who engage in sex live longer than those who avoid such activity.

"Sexuality can revitalize and energize your life," I tell patients who ask for bold, to-the-point answers on the subject. "Consenting adults who engage in sex often look and feel better, and my experience has shown that seniors who enjoy physical intimacy generally live longer."

Some doctors including homeopaths have labeled sexuality as a profound energy that produces, prolongs and energizes human life. Those who embrace such a philosophy should consider making quality sex and quality sleep among the priorities of their lives.

16
Closing Comments

Without exaggeration, I consider anyone who has completed this guidebook as extremely fortunate or perhaps even "lucky."

As you might very well imagine, a vast majority of people lack the basic and essential sleep-related information you have just reviewed.

By this point many readers likely realize that many people who lack this information likely face an increased probability of experiencing severe health issues.

"To sleep, perchance to dream," says the famed age-old saying first penned by the legendary bard William Shakespeare in "Hamlet."

Rest assured, throughout the remainder of my life I'll stay dedicated and energized to help more patients get this critical information to as many people as possible who might benefit.

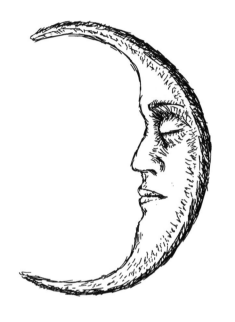

About the Author

James W. Forsythe, M.D., H.M.D., has long been considered one of the most respected physicians in the United States, particularly for his treatment of cancer and the legal use of human growth hormone. In the mid-1960s, Dr. Forsythe graduated with honors from University California at Berkeley and earned his Medical Degree from University of California, San Francisco, before spending two years residency in Pathology at Tripler Army Hospital, Honolulu. After a tour of duty in Vietnam, he returned to San Francisco and completed an internal medicine residency and an oncology fellowship. He is also a world-renowned speaker and author. He has co-authored, been mentioned in and/or written chapters in bestsellers. To name a few: "An Alternative Medicine Definitive Guide to Cancer;" "Knockout, Interviews with Doctors who are Curing Cancer" Suzanne Somers' number one bestseller; "The Ultimate Guide To Natural Health, Quick Reference A-Z Directory of Natural Remedies for Diseases and Ailments;" "Anti-Aging Cures;" "The Healing Power of Sleep;" "Outsmart Your Cancer: Alternative Non-Toxic Treatments That Work" and "Compassionate Oncology ~ What Conventional Cancer Specialists Don't Want You To Know;" and "Obaminable Care," "Complete Pain," "Natural Pain Killers," and "Your Secret to the Fountain of Youth ~ What They Don't Want You to Know About HGH Human Growth Hormone," "Take Control of Your Cancer," and the "Emergency Radiation Medical Handbook."

Contact Information

Century Wellness Clinic, 521 Hammill Lane

Reno, NV, 89511

(775) 827-0707

RenoWellnessDr@Yahoo.com